REDISCOVERING CHILDHOOD TRAUMA

HISTORICAL CASEBOOK

AND

CLINICAL APPLICATIONS

Clinical Practice

Number 28

Judith H. Gold, M.D., F.R.C.P.C.
Series Editor

REDISCOVERING CHILDHOOD TRAUMA

HISTORICAL CASEBOOK AND CLINICAL APPLICATIONS

Edited by

Jean M. Goodwin, M.D., M.P.H.

Professor, Department of Psychiatry
and Behavioral Sciences
University of Texas Medical School
Galveston, Texas

American Psychiatric Press, Inc.

Washington, DC
London, England

Note: The authors have worked to ensure that all information in this book concerning drug dosages, schedules, and routes of administration is accurate as of the time of publication and consistent with standards set by the U.S. Food and Drug Administration and the general medical community. As medical research and practice advance, however, therapeutic standards may change. For this reason and because human and mechanical errors sometimes occur, we recommend that readers follow the advice of a physician who is directly involved in their care or the care of a member of their family.

Manufactured in the United States of America on acid-free paper
First Edition 96 95 94 93 4 3 2 1

American Psychiatric Press, Inc.
1400 K Street, N.W., Washington, DC 20005

Library of Congress Cataloging-in-Publication Data

Rediscovering childhood trauma : historical casebook and clinical applications / [edited by] Jean M. Goodwin. — 1st ed.
p. cm. — (Clinical practice series, no. 28)
Includes bibliographical references and index.
ISBN 0-88048-460-8 (alk. paper)
1. Adult child abuse victims—Mental health. 2. Adult child abuse victims—Case studies. 3. Psychic trauma in children—Case studies. 4. Post-traumatic stress disorder—Case studies. I. Goodwin, Jean, 1946– . II. Series: Clinical practice, no. 28.
[DNLM: 1. Child Abuse—psychology. 2. Mythology. 3. Psychoanalysis—history. 4. Psychoanalytic Interpretation. 5. Stress Disorders, Post-Traumatic—in infancy & childhood. W1 CL767J no. 28 / WS 350.5 R317]
RC569.5.C55R43 1993
616.85′8369—dc20
DNLM/DLC
for Library of Congress 92-17706
CIP

British Library Cataloguing in Publication Data

A CIP record is available from the British Library.

Contents

Contributors

Catherine Fine, Ph.D.
Program Coordinator, Dissociative Disorders Program, The Institute of Pennsylvania Hospital, Philadelphia, Pennsylvania; Clinical Assistant Professor of Psychiatry, Temple University School of Medicine, Philadelphia, Pennsylvania

Jean M. Goodwin, M.D., M.P.H.
Professor, Department of Psychiatry and Behavioral Sciences, University of Texas Medical School, Galveston, Texas

Sally Hill, M.S.W.
Doctoral Candidate, Chicago Institute for Clinical Social Work, Chicago, Illinois

Richard P. Kluft, M.D.
Clinical Professor of Psychiatry, Temple University School of Medicine; Director, Dissociative Disorders Program, The Institute of Pennsylvania Hospital, Philadelphia, Pennsylvania

Kathryn C. Krieg, M.D.
Assistant Professor; Medical Director, Managed Care; and Associate Director, Undergraduate Education, Department of Psychiatry and Mental Health Sciences, Medical College of Wisconsin, Milwaukee, Wisconsin

Richard J. Loewenstein, M.D.
Senior Psychiatrist and Director, Dissociative Disorders Programs, Sheppard and Enoch Pratt Hospital; Assistant Clinical Professor, Department of Psychiatry and Behavioral Science, University of Maryland School of Medicine, Baltimore, Maryland

Barbara J. Murray, M.D.
Private Practice, Suncoast Medical Clinics, St. Petersburg, Florida

Jeffrey Richards, M.D.
Psychiatric Resident, U.S. Air Force Hospital, Lackland Air Force Base, San Antonio, Texas

Kenneth X. Robbins, M.D.
Attending Psychiatrist, Department of Psychiatry, Alexandria Hospital, Alexandria, Virginia; Consultant, Department of Psychiatry and Neurology, Walter Reed Army Medical Center, Washington, DC

Onno van der Hart, Ph.D.
Chief, Trauma and Dissociation Team, Regional Institute of Ambulatory Mental Health Care (RIAGG) South/New West, Amsterdam, Netherlands

Eliezer Witztum, M.D.
Jerusalem Mental Health Center—Ezrath Nashim, Jerusalem, Israel

Introduction

to the Clinical Practice Series

Over the years of its existence the series of monographs entitled *Clinical Insights* gradually became focused on providing current, factual, and theoretical material of interest to the clinician working outside of a hospital setting. To reflect this orientation, the name of the Series has been changed to *Clinical Practice.*

The Clinical Practice Series will provide books that give the mental health clinician a practical, clinical approach to a variety of psychiatric problems. These books will provide up-to-date literature reviews and emphasize the most recent treatment methods. Thus, the publications in the Series will interest clinicians working both in psychiatry and in the other mental health professions.

Each year a number of books will be published dealing with all aspects of clinical practice. In addition, from time to time when appropriate, the publications may be revised and updated. Thus, the Series will provide quick access to relevant and important areas of psychiatric practice. Some books in the Series will be authored by a person considered to be an expert in that particular area; others will be edited by such an expert, who will also draw together other knowledgeable authors to produce a comprehensive overview of that topic.

Some of the books in the Clinical Practice Series will have their foundation in presentations at an annual meeting of the American Psychiatric Association. All will contain the most recently available information on the subjects discussed. Theoretical and scientific data will be applied to clinical situations, and case illustrations will be utilized in order to make the material even more relevant for the practitioner. Thus, the Clinical Practice Series should provide educational reading in a compact format especially designed for the mental health clinician–psychiatrist.

Judith H. Gold, M.D., F.R.C.P.C.
Series Editor
Clinical Practice Series

Clinical Practice Series Titles

Treating Chronically Mentally Ill Women (#1)
Edited by Leona L. Bachrach, Ph.D., and Carol C. Nadelson, M.D.

Divorce as a Developmental Process (#2)
Edited by Judith H. Gold, M.D., F.R.C.P.C.

Family Violence: Emerging Issues of a National Crisis (#3)
Edited by Leah J. Dickstein, M.D., and Carol C. Nadelson, M.D.

Anxiety and Depressive Disorders in the Medical Patient (#4)
By Leonard R. Derogatis, Ph.D., and Thomas N. Wise, M.D.

Anxiety: New Findings for the Clinician (#5)
Edited by Peter Roy-Byrne, M.D.

The Neuroleptic Malignant Syndrome and Related Conditions (#6)
By Arthur Lazarus, M.D., Stephan C. Mann, M.D., and Stanley N. Caroff, M.D.

Juvenile Homicide (#7)
Edited by Elissa P. Benedek, M.D., and Dewey G. Cornell, Ph.D.

Measuring Mental Illness: Psychometric Assessment for Clinicians (#8)
Edited by Scott Wetzler, Ph.D.

Family Involvement in Treatment of the Frail Elderly (#9)
Edited by Marion Zucker Goldstein, M.D.

Psychiatric Care of Migrants: A Clinical Guide (#10)
By Joseph Westermeyer, M.D., M.P.H., Ph.D.

Office Treatment of Schizophrenia (#11)
Edited by Mary V. Seeman, M.D., F.R.C.P.C., and Stanley E. Greben, M.D., F.R.C.P.C.

The Psychosocial Impact of Job Loss (#12)
By Nick Kates, M.B.B.S., F.R.C.P.C., Barrie S. Greiff, M.D., and Duane Q. Hagen, M.D.

New Perspectives on Narcissism (#13)
Edited by Eric M. Plakun, M.D.

Clinical Management of Gender Identity Disorders in Children and Adults (#14)
Edited by Ray Blanchard, Ph.D., and Betty W. Steiner, M.B., F.R.C.P.C.

Family Approaches in Treatment of Eating Disorders (#15)
Edited by D. Blake Woodside, M.D., M.Sc., F.R.C.P.C., and Lorie Shekter-Wolfson, M.S.W., C.S.W.

Adolescent Psychotherapy (#16)
Edited by Marcia Slomowitz, M.D.

Benzodiazepines in Clinical Practice: Risks and Benefits (#17)
Edited by Peter P. Roy-Byrne, M.D., and Deborah S. Cowley, M.D.

Current Treatments of Obsessive-Compulsive Disorder (#18)
Edited by Michele Tortora Pato, M.D., and Joseph Zohar, M.D.

Children and AIDS (#19)
Edited by Margaret L. Stuber, M.D.

Special Problems in Managing Eating Disorders (#20)
Edited by Joel Yager, M.D., Harry E. Gwirtsman, M.D., and Carole K. Edelstein, M.D.

Suicide and Clinical Practice (#21)
Edited by Douglas Jacobs, M.D.

Anxiety Disorders in Children and Adolescents (#22)
By Syed Arshad Husain, M.D., F.R.C.P.C., F.R.C.Psych., and Javad Kashani, M.D.

Psychopharmacological Treatment Complications in the Elderly (#23)
Edited by Charles A. Shamoian, M.D., Ph.D.

Responding to Disaster: A Guide for Mental Health Professionals (#24)
Edited by Linda S. Austin, M.D.

Psychiatric Aspects of Symptom Management in Cancer Patients (#25)
Edited by William Breitbart, M.D., and Jimmie C. Holland, M.D.

Sexuality, Reproduction, and Long-Term Mental Illness (#26)
Edited by Roberta J. Apfel, M.D., M.P.H., and Maryellen H. Handel, Ph.D.

Treatment of Adult Survivors of Incest (#27)
Edited by Patricia L. Paddison, M.D.

Rediscovering Childhood Trauma: Historical Casebook and Clinical Applications (#28)
Edited by Jean M. Goodwin, M.D., M.P.H.

Foreword

On Paradigms and the Legitimization of Myopia

The importance of exogenous and intentionally inflicted trauma for the development of subsequent psychopathology is increasingly appreciated (Kluft 1990a). The scope of humanity's proclivity for the abuse and exploitation of those unable to defend themselves against such depredations often seems matched only by the ardor with which the ubiquity of such behaviors is denied, minimized, and rationalized. It is all too easy to dismiss accounts of mistreatment or to view them with skepticism. It is tempting to disbelieve what is distressing to hear and disquieting to contemplate. As Goodwin (1985) noted: "Incredulity can be understood as an intellectualized variant of derealization; and, like the dissociative defenses, incredulity is an effective way to gain distance from terrifying realities" (p. 7).

The impact of trauma is far more pervasive than would be expected from a tabulation of the prevalence of those conditions that are understood to be wholly or predominantly posttraumatic in origin. Those who have been mistreated may manifest a wide variety of symptoms, syndromes, and character traits that may not initially be appreciated as "disguised presentations" (a term introduced by Gelinas [1983] in the incest literature) of what has befallen them. Complex and puzzling behavior patterns with no consciously appreciated connection with the past may remain the only landmarks of the ongoing impact of overwhelming events (Blank 1985). A history of childhood traumatization may make conditions not usually associated with such antecedents more difficult to treat (R. Schultz, B. Braun, R. P. Kluft, unpublished data, October 1985) and is highly correlated with problems and misadventures in the course of psychotherapeutic treatments (Kluft 1989, 1990b).

Rediscovering Childhood Trauma offers penetrating insights into myths, people, and classic psychiatric cases that have already been studied quite thoughtfully from a variety of perspectives. Viewed with considerations of trauma in mind, these cases often seem less grand and less fascinating. They are no longer beautiful illustrations of brilliant minds at work and stimulating studies of important theories actualized and exemplified; they become embarrassing texts for the consideration of the lengths to which psychiatric models and theories go to discount the dark underside of the human character. They become not only important historical accounts and crucial demonstrations of the soaring intellects and facile theorizing of those who attempt to explain them, but they also stand as reminders that many an explanation or idea is so striking and initially compelling because it has excluded (or never considered) countervailing data, has protected its pristine luster by failing to become more battle-scarred and humbled in the rarely successful effort to eliminate alternative possible explanations, is presented in a manner that detracts attention from its blemishes and shortcomings, and may reduce anxiety by protecting its adherents from unsettling and overstimulating materials.

It is interesting to contemplate why historical cases continue to exert a fascination and to inspire reinterpretations. One obvious reason is that the more we learn, the more perspectives and insights we have to offer. That this occurs and will continue to occur is inevitable. However, there must be more that governs this process than the expansion of knowledge per se, because many reinterpretations are based on materials and concepts that were available previously, but for some reason(s) were omitted from consideration or overlooked.

The subjects and central concerns of this book are a case in point. The realization that trauma is not a good thing is hardly novel. Janet was quite aware of the deleterious impact of trauma, as was Freud. Although Freud repudiated the seduction theory and developed alternative models, he was ever mindful of the impact of noxious events. Yet the role of exogenous trauma in most forms of psychopathology was minimized for several generations. Furthermore, even in ancient texts, the impact of trauma is often bypassed as the text focuses on another theme. To illustrate, one might turn to the Biblical account of the binding and near-sacrifice of Isaac by Abraham. Clearly the major theme is the obedience of Abraham to the word of God, because he was willing to sacrifice his only son at God's behest. Perhaps the readers of this book will notice the Bible's neglect of the traumatic impact of this pivotal event upon Isaac.

Other ancient texts offer a more realistic perspective. In Virgil's *Aeneid,* a wonderful scene occurs among the dead in the underworld.

They are offered the opportunity to choose the souls in which they will be reincarnated. There is a great rush for those that augur lives of fame and fortune and wealth. However, Odysseus, the wiliest of men, looks elsewhere. As the others seek to "improve their lot," so does he. With great vigor and purpose, informed by the wisdom of a man who has been a great leader, chieftain, and adventurer, tempest-tossed, battle-hardened, who "has seen it all," he seeks out and claims the soul of a man of moderate means and fortunes, free from the perils and turmoils of poverty and deprivation on the one hand and of the dangers and stresses of riches, power, and renown on the other. This early and presumably apocryphal tale is only a single case study (or single legend surmise), but it is remarkably consistent with the modern appreciation that stress and trauma, while inevitable, are not terribly desirable.

We must ask and explore the question: why must childhood trauma be rediscovered? Why does what is known become peripheral, even disregarded, over the course of time? Is it possible that as we advance in our knowledge we pay a price, and is that price the neglect or impoverishment of some areas of understanding in connection with the gains made in others? Does something happen so that we are condemned to forget what we know and periodically are forced to remind ourselves of this? What of the dreadful impact it has upon the integrity of what is called scientific progress and upon the quality of the patient care that we render?

The answer to the uncomfortable question of should childhood trauma be rediscovered appears to be affirmative. There exists within the very nature of the process of scientific progress a series of mechanisms that legitimizes myopic and scotomatic intellectual vision and encourages absolute antiscience in the name of keener insight into the nature of a particular branch of science's subjects of inquiry. That psychiatry managed to accord minimal attention to various forms of familial violence and their sequela for a protracted period of time does not indict the profession. However, it does warn that progress, like any powerful intervention, is not without some undesirable side effects. It also serves as a cautionary warning that every science must arrange to monitor itself lest the ideas that are au courant lead to the disregard or disavowal of what is known and important, but is not in the center of the field's concern at a given point of time.

The story is told of the policeman who, while walking his beat late one night, came up to a corner lamppost and found a man nearby, somewhat the worse for drink, searching the ground on his hands and knees. The policeman asked the man what he was looking for, and the man said that he had dropped his car keys and could not go home until he found them. Eager to be of assistance, the officer joined the man and searched the area meticulously. When he was sure that the keys were not to be found, the policeman asked the man if he were sure that he had dropped the keys where they were searching. The man quickly responded that he had lost the keys half a block away. Perplexed, the officer asked, "Then why, if you lost the keys down the block, are you crawling around on your hands and knees under the lamppost?" Without hesitation, the man rejoined, "Well you see, officer, it's too dark over there!" In many ways this scenario speaks to why a book like *Rediscovering Childhood Trauma* is timely, if not overdue. All too often, science deals with what is under the lamppost and fails to look down the block where the keys were lost.

In his classic study *The Structure of Scientific Revolutions,* Kuhn (1970) points out that the course of scientific progress is not continuous, additive, and linear. At a given point in time, a science is governed by a paradigm, which is an advance, idea, or an experiment that will "define the legitimate problems and methods and research in a field for succeeding generations. . . . The achievement [is] sufficiently open-ended to leave all sorts of problems for the redefined group of practitioners to solve" (Kuhn 1970, p. 10). The definition of what is scientific is determined by the scope of the paradigm, not by data and proof alone. Moreover, a scientific revolution is described not as an integration of the old and the new, but as "a non-cumulative developmental episode in which an older paradigm is replaced in whole or in part by an incompatible new one" (p. 91).

Perception is grossly altered by shifts in paradigms:

> During revolutions scientists see new and different things when looking with familiar instruments in places they have looked before. . . . In so far as their only recourse to that world is what they see and do, we may want to say that after a revolution scientists are responding to a different world. (Kuhn 1970, p. 111)

This leads, inevitably, to clashes between those who embrace different paradigms.

> The proponents of competing paradigms practice their trades in different worlds. . . . The two groups . . . see different things when they look at the same point in the same direction . . . what they look at has not changed. But in some areas they see different things, and they see them in different relations one to the other. That is why a law that cannot even be demonstrated to one group of scientists may occasionally seem intuitively obvious to another. Equally, it is why, before they can hope to communicate fully, one group or the other must experience the conversion that we have been calling a paradigm shift. Just because it is a transition between incommensurables, the transition between the competing paradigms cannot be made a step at a time, forced by logic and neutral experience. Like the gestalt switch, it must occur all at once (though not necessarily in an instant) or not at all. (Kuhn 1970, p. 150)

Among groups of psychiatrists embracing different paradigms, it is commonplace to hear anecdotes that demonstrate the wisdom of one paradigm over another. Biologically oriented psychiatrists regale themselves with tales of patients who did not improve in years of psychotherapy yet had dramatic relief with medications.

Psychotherapeutically oriented practitioners enjoy accounts in which years were wasted in exhausting the entire pharmacopoeia upon a patient with little more than side effects to show for the endeavor, whereupon the patient improved once a crucial issue was worked through. Many who point to the crucial importance of trauma tell of cases in which years of unproductive treatment had failed to identify and address the trauma, followed by significant or total improvement once its importance had been acknowledged and dealt with. We are all more inclined to report and dwell upon our successes than our failures.

There are many consequences to the type of scientific change that Kuhn (1970) has described. The embracing of a paradigm means the redefinition of what is scientific and a redetermination of what is the proper study of that particular branch of science in which the paradigm prevails. What may be genuine and crucial, but does not fall within the paradigm, may be declared beyond the pale of true science. The risk of intellectual totalitarianism is inherent in paradigm shifts. Perhaps psychiatry has benefited by the weakness of its paradigms; considerable diversity has been retained, and no one paradigm has ever completely effaced the others. However, should the adherents of one paradigm dominate academia and/or the funding streams that nourish research, this could become possible. Certainly, the power of advocates of biological psychiatry has not been beneficial to those whose research addresses issues of great importance but which may be seen as less worthy by those in biologically oriented research, because it does not embrace the paradigm by which they define what is scientific (i.e., become illuminated under the lamppost of psychobiology under which they search!).

Intellectual arrogance and deprecation of what is foreign to a paradigm of choice are hardly beneficial for the advancement of knowledge. Furthermore, by discrediting alternative explanations, there is the risk that a science will attempt to proceed by accumulating data that are consistent with a paradigm of choice and that it will become solipsistic rather than integrated with other bodies of knowledge. Reasoning by accumulating instances of confirmation (enumerative inductionalism) is less demanding than thinking that insists that alternative hypotheses be considered and eliminated by the weight of evidence (eliminative inductionalism). The risk of scientific myopia and scotomatization is considerable.

Why, again, do we need to rediscover trauma and to study new instances in which theories and insights have been drawn from situations with definite or likely traumatic components that have not been taken into consideration? We must do so because we are expanding our knowledge of trauma and its impact, and we can gain by applying our new understanding. We must do so because we *Homo sapiens* are adept at blocking out our appreciation of the existence and sequelae of trauma. We must do so because major prevailing paradigms systematically distract our attention from the importance of trauma. Because we have been educated within the myopia of these paradigms, they hinder our perception of events from the perspective of trauma.

If we understand the perspective of trauma theory as offering a new and important paradigm, we can hope to learn from what Kuhn (1970) and others have discovered and take steps to refrain from creating a literature that dismisses and disdains alternative perspectives. Those who study trauma appreciate its adverse impact on the integration of not only the individual but also the entire familial, social, and societal network within which the trauma occurs. As a group, these researchers are making efforts to bring these realizations to bear upon the intellectual climate to which they are contributing. The authors in *Rediscovering Childhood Trauma* have not made an effort to discount what has gone before; they clearly wish to complement, supplement, and enrich what they have inherited.

Consideration of the perspective of trauma and its impact is an essential component of the informed assessment and treatment of the psychiatric patient. It is as necessary as a mental status exam, a descriptive diagnosis, a developmental and family history, a psychodynamic formulation, and the ordering of appropriate laboratory and other studies. It is unfortunate that a history of significant trauma is highly prevalent in psychiatric populations, but it is still more unfortunate that the elicitation of such histories is not.

Discussing trauma with patients is still far from routine. It is not unusual for veteran patients who have been through many treatments and hospital stays to comment, when such information is requested, that they have never been asked such questions before.

By making us aware of the missing dimensions of the cases and constructs that we have studied and with which we are already familiar, Dr. Goodwin and her collaborators sensitize us to consider and compel us to search out the possibility that the patients we see, who embody so much of what is described and demonstrated in this book, are the contemporary victims of unsuspected or unacknowledged trauma. The discovery of the connection between what may have been previously refractory symptoms and traumatic events often can turn a frustrating or stalemated treatment into a process that can bring about impressive growth and change. It may prevent a patient from becoming a treatment failure by virtue of having received a therapy that failed to address a basic aspect of that patient's disturbance, regardless of the presenting symptoms. Many previously refractory patients with the phenotypic appearance of disorders not usually associated with trauma will be found to be manifesting disguised presentations of trauma that now become accessible to treatment (Gelinas 1983). The patient who is correctly understood is more likely to benefit from treatment than the patient who is not. An essential aspect of the search for understanding is the correction of the perceptual distortions and blind spots that are inherent in our paradigms and in their clashes. Our patients deserve no less.

Richard P. Kluft, M.D.

References

Blank AS: The unconscious flashback to the war in Vietnam veterans: clinical mystery, legal defense, and community problem, in The Trauma of War: Stress and Recovery in Vietnam Veterans. Edited by Sonnenberg SM, Blank AS, Talbott JA. Washington, DC, American Psychiatric Press, 1985, pp 293–308

Gelinas D: The persisting negative effects of incest. Psychiatry 46:312–332, 1983

Goodwin JM: Credibility problems in multiple personality disorder and abused children, in Childhood Antecedents of Multiple Personality. Edited by Kluft RP. Washington, DC, American Psychiatric Press, 1985, pp 21–35

Kluft RP: Treating the patient who has been sexually exploited by a prior psychotherapist. Psychiatr Clin North Am 12:483–500, 1989

Kluft RP (ed): Incest-Related Syndromes of Adult Psychopathology. Washington, DC, American Psychiatric Press, 1990a

Kluft RP: Incest and subsequent revictimization: the case of therapist-patient sexual exploitation, with a description of the sitting duck syndrome, in Incest-Related Syndromes of Adult Psychopathology. Edited by Kluft RP. Washington, DC, American Psychiatric Press, 1990b, pp 263–287

Kuhn TS: The Structure of Scientific Revolutions, 2nd Edition, Enlarged. Chicago, IL, University of Chicago Press, 1970

Preface

This book began as an idea for a symposium for the 1989 annual meeting of the American Psychiatric Association in San Francisco. For many years I had used and borrowed historical examples to explain and illustrate the posttraumatic symptoms that follow child abuse. By the summer of 1988, I realized that these examples were accumulating to a degree that warranted collection. The idea was to pair each historical case with present-day clinical material in order to highlight the clinical lessons in each case. Some chapters grew out of that symposium: Oedipus, Electra, Mary Reynolds and Estelle, Anna O, Dora, and *Rose Garden.* What my collaborators and I noted as we worked on these materials is that they were helpful not only as rhetorical aids but also as vehicles for clarifying clinical concepts and for broadening professional dialogue about childhood trauma and its interactions with other mental processes.

The rhetorical points to be made are that both childhood trauma and the severe symptom complexes that follow it have existed throughout history. They appear new to us today only because we have been so deft at avoiding, ignoring, and minimizing such histories.

In these historical cases, one can only speculate about childhood trauma; substantiation is no longer possible. With mythical figures like Oedipus and Electra, we are operating entirely within the realm of ideas and imagination. What we can notice however about psychiatry's reaction to these myths is that the extensive family histories of homicidal violence have seldom been connected causally to the severe symptoms described in both protagonists. In one sense, the inconclusiveness of the historical cases is salutary. It would be folly to suggest today, as Freud did 100 years ago, that each time we see certain severe symptoms, these must be the result of childhood trauma. What the historical cases suggest is that this is one possibility to consider. We can begin to ask how psychiatrists could tell the story of Freud's 17th-century painter while leaving out the Thirty Years' War or tell the story of Mary Reynolds while omitting the Birmingham Riots. Psychiatry seems to postulate that terrorization by death threat, physical pain, and loss are rather weak explanations for psychological developments in children and must be replaced by something more real or profound. In the case of the Marquis de Sade, we are looking not so much at his own symptoms as sequelae of childhood trauma (although that question is asked) as at the fact that the Marquis existed and that his impact as a trauma vector for child victims must have been devastating.

Freud, of course, was a master at using history to make his points in a way so convincing as to overwhelm opposition. I hope these cases do more than that. They provide extensive clinical data, sometimes including lifetime follow-up. They allow us to recognize similar clinical pathology in a variety of cultural and historical contexts. They present to us novel treatment interventions, some of which are no longer extant or ethical. They force us to be clear about the theoretical differences between ourselves and clinicians who have analyzed the same materials in the past. This last point is important, because excessive polarization between trauma theory and psychodynamic theory has produced many clinicians with solid grounding in only one of the two perspectives.

As the term in used in this book, trauma is defined psychodynamically, as an event that overwhelms the defensive capacities of the child. The details of such events are sought because they tend to be forgotten and because their immediate and long-term impacts are serious, but also because they shape the child's subsequent fantasies, fears, and wishes about the event and the lessons the child draws about its meaning. This book, although it introduces interpretations based on trauma theory, forces the reader to review previous approaches to the historical materials that involved only intrapsychic or drive explanations. With several theories on the table, we are a step closer to where we need to be. Ultimately we must integrate the understanding of trauma and its impact into a more comprehensive grasp of how the child's internal representational world develops in relation to the interpersonal world.

There are two basic approaches to reading this book. One can read straight through, savoring the chronology and observing the variations in posttraumatic phenomenology illustrated in each historical case; or one can focus on a particular clinical problem and locate the chapters relevant to that clinical issue. The introduction to the section containing the chapter of clinical interest will give the reader an orientation to historical context and theoretical relevance.

For the reader, this book can provide a journey through time and through a complex syndrome of symptoms. For the editor, this book has also meant journeys through geography and within relationships. My thanks go to friends and strangers who welcomed me to Delphi, Athens, Paris, Meadville, Vienna, and Chestnut Lodge, and especially to David Feinsilver, Ann-Louise Silver, and Dexter Bullard, Jr., at the Lodge.

Coauthors and contributors more often edited me than I them, and to my great benefit. Richard P. Kluft supported the project from before its beginnings and listened to drafts in the early days before they existed on paper. I am grateful to Judy Herman, Reina Attias, Marion Tolpin, and Julie Dunleavy, who kindly read parts of the manuscript in draft form and encouraged me to talk about the project. Kimberly James-Jones was invaluable in keeping the manuscripts, correspondence, and computer files straight. My thanks go also to Rod McVeety, who helped with the introduction to Chapter 9.

I am most grateful to my husband and children who have been generous in sharing me not only with my real patients, but also with these patients from the past who I can care for only in the clinic of my imagination.

Jean M. Goodwin, M.D., M.P.H.

Section I

Mythical Figures and Psychoanalytic Paradigms

Of all peoples the Greeks have dreamed the dream of life best.
Goethe, *Iphigenie auf Tauris*

It seems clearly probable that myths are distorted vestiges of the wish fulfillments of whole nations.
Sigmund Freud, "Creative Writers and Daydreaming"
Standard Edition, Volume 9

Myths are to answer the awkward questions children ask.
Robert Graves, *The Greek Myths*

I come to give you something and the gift is my own beaten self;
no feast for the eyes; yet in me is more lasting grace than beauty.
Sophocles
Oedipus at Colonus

Editor's Introduction

Why do psychiatrists continue to study Oedipus and Electra? Why include them here as cases? There is no good evidence they were even human beings, one might argue, much less sufferers of any particular pathology.

However, the Greeks seem to think of them as people. When one goes to Delphi, the guide shows you the triple crossroads where Oedipus slew his father, Laius. At Mycenae, one is shown Agamemnon's death mask, the golden impression of those features Electra grieved over so unceasingly. Medieval scholars developed complex concordances relating the dates of mythologic heroes to those of biblical characters (Veyne 1988). Freud, too, seemed to think of Oedipus and Electra as people and followed avidly the archaeological explorations of his contemporary Heinrich Schliemann, who spent his career digging wherever he sensed that Homer had told him to dig, working from the hypothesis that all those stories were true and all those characters were real people.

Whether we see them as dreams, wish-fulfillments, moral fables, or as biographies of real people polished to immortality through the art of wonderful storytellers, one cannot deny that the stories of Oedipus and Electra are gifts among the finest handed down to us by the Greeks, and enduring sources of insight into the human condition.

In literature, these myths are used to illustrate the fatal flaw—that intrinsic paradox in human nature whereby our most vital survival skills become simultaneously the agency of our self-destruction. This is most clear for Oedipus, whose cleverness is the source of his power. When the Oracle at Delphi dooms him to kill his parents, he counters by leaving the country. He outwits not only the oracle but later the dreaded Sphinx; he alone is able to decipher her riddle. (Freud identified with Oedipus the riddlesolver, especially when immersed in solving the riddle of dreams. Not only did Freud speak of Oedipus at those times as if he were a real person but also as if that real person might be Freud himself [Anzieu 1986]). The prize Oedipus wins for decoding the riddle is the surrounding kingdom and its queen, Jocasta. So, years later, when his kingdom is threatened by a plague, Oedipus is determined to unravel the murder mystery said by soothsayers to have caused the plague, despite good advice from all sides that he should desist. Now, finally, his cleverness undoes him and turns out not to have been the engine of his previous good fortune either. Oedipus learns that the parents he so protectively left were only adoptive. A rude and brutal traveler that he killed incidentally on the road was his natural father, and the queen won by his riddlesolving was his mother.

The resulting disaster is complete. Jocasta hangs herself; Oedipus, sentenced to exile, blinds himself. To dismantle his pernicious cleverness? To protect himself from the guilt-provoking sight of the surrounding disaster? To shift his gaze from the outer world to the inner? To punish himself by symbolic castration? All have been suggested by scholars who keep forgetting that Oedipus is not really even a person and who keep finding themselves involved as intensely with his misfortunes as they are with their own.

Electra's fatal flaw is her unrelenting hatred of her mother and thirst for vengeance. The problem is not that Electra's complaints are unjust. Clytemnestra did conspire with her lover Aegisthus to kill Electra's father Agamemnon; Clytemnestra did indeed exile Electra's brother Orestes and has effectively disinherited Electra. The problem that Electra does not see is that her murderous and implacable refusal to forgive and her self-righteous bitterness are exact reflections of everything that she hates in Clytemnestra. Also, for years, the only victim of Electra's obsessive revenge plotting is herself. It is she and not Clytemnestra who is wasting away, losing friends, cutting herself off from merriment and fun. In the end, however, having acquired allies, Electra successfully executes her revenge, despite her guilty misgivings; and, unlike her brother, she escapes punishment. Electra goes on to marry suitably, just as she had longed to do. Unfortunately, we do not have a surviving play about Electra's middle age to tell us whether the vindictiveness that had served her so well in youth simply evaporated once her problem with Clytemnestra was solved, or whether it remained to become an internal adversary (Blundell 1989).

Freud took the Oedipus story and made it into the Oedipus complex. According to Freud (1900/1962), the fate that Oedipus could not escape was the universal wish to marry the parent of the opposite gender and the consequent murderous rivalry with the parent of the same sex. Jung (1915/1961) suggested Electra as a good example of the female version of this configuration.

What was left out in these analyses was the violence. Oedipus was not an ordinary little boy. He was a little boy whose father was a pedophile and whose parents did not make love except when the husband was drunk. He was a little boy whose father planned to kill him even before he was born and who executed the attempt with maximum cruelty. When Laius sent the infant Oedipus off to be exposed to die alone on a mountainside, he first passed an iron rod behind both of the baby's Achilles tendons in order to cripple him (Ross 1982).

Years later, when a rude passerby ran his chariot over the still-crippled foot of young Oedipus, some stories say that Oedipus went wild with rage, perhaps triggered by somatic memories of the unremembered and unrememberable infantile abuse, and killed the man (who turned out the be Laius himself and not merely a revenant) after first dispatching all his adversary's servants (Edmunds 1985). (Laius was never one to get involved in a fair fight but made certain the odds were in his favor.)

It was perhaps because Oedipus still walked with a staff because of his foot mutilation that he knew how to solve the riddle of the Sphinx: "What walks on four feet at morning, two at noon, and three at evening?" Oedipus had put a lot of thought into feet and was already walking with "three"; and, as with so many abused children grown up, his development had been so distorted as to make him as much of a patchwork chimera of developmental stages as was his adversary, the Sphinx. Parts of Oedipus had remained infantile, parts were adult, and some parts were ancient, having grown old too soon in order to cope with the life-threatening abuse (Michels 1986).

We are reminded again of modern-day trauma victims with dissociative disorders as we watch Oedipus having so much difficulty piecing together his life story, once he is forced to try. The fatal fight with his father in particular seems to keep going out of focus for Oedipus and disappearing from his functional memory. His angry impulsiveness is also a familiar aspect of abuse victims and continues to the end of his life, when one of his last acts is to renew the fatal curse he has placed on his own sons. The one thing Oedipus has learned through long experience and suffering by the time he dies at Colonus is that he cannot control everything. The story seems to say that this is wisdom enough (Felman 1987).

Electra also is not an ordinary little girl. She is a little girl whose father has killed some of her mother's babies, and vice versa. Her mother has killed her father and has attempted to kill her brother Orestes. Electra's sister will die by suicide. Electra is a survivor in the literal sense, but a survivor who suffers symptoms. She is depressed and talks of suicide. She has cut her hair and no longer tries to look pretty. Like Cinderella, she is barred from parties and dances. Electra complains all the time, and people no longer like to be around her. She prefers to withdraw, in any case, because her revenge fantasies have become the most alive part of her life.

The following chapters pursue this latter aspect of the old Greek stories—the violence toward the children—and ask what the myths can tell us about modern-day patients who come to us ostensibly with individual emotional problems but who are also refugees from violent families. This perspective invites us to look at our theories in a new way as well. From the vantage of trauma theory, what the Oedipus complex describes is a situation in early childhood of crisis, conflict, and negative emotion. This situation is resolved by identification, by amnesia, and by developing a new moral agency. What if this happens every time the multiply abused child is overwhelmed? This is one way to understand the development of multiple personality disorder, with its multiple unintegrated identifications and moral stances kept apart by massive amnesia.

Although the trauma recovery approach is emphasized in this book, it does not, in my view, detract from any of the older approaches. Oedipus and Electra deal not only with their violent parents and violent pasts but also with their own fatal flaws and with longings and fears that go far beyond those that they can allow themselves to know.

References

Anzieu D: Freud's Self-Analysis. Madison, CT, International Universities Press, 1986

Blundell MW: Helping Friends and Harming Enemies: A Study in Sophocles and Greek Ethics. New York, Cambridge University Press, 1989

Edmunds L: Oedipus: The Ancient Legend and Its Later Analogues. Baltimore, MD, Johns Hopkins University Press, 1985

Felman S: Beyond Oedipus: the specimen story of psychoanalysis, in Jacques Lacan and the Adventure of Insight: Psychoanalysis and Contemporary Culture. Edited by Felman S. Cambridge, MA, Harvard University Press, 1987, pp 99–160

Freud S: The interpretation of dreams (1900), in The Standard Edition of the Complete Works of Sigmund Freud, Vols 4 and 5. Edited and translated by Strachey J. London, Hogarth Press, 1962

Jung K: The theory of psychoanalysis (1915), in The Collected Works of C.G. Jung, Vol 4. New York, Bollingen Foundation, 1961

Michels R: Oedipus and insight. Psychoanal Q 55:599–617, 1986

Ross JM: Oedipus revisited: Laius and the "Laius complex." Psychoanal Study Child 37:169–200, 1982

Veyne P: Did the Greeks Believe in Their Myths? Chicago, IL, University of Chicago Press, 1988

Chapter 1

Oedipus: Uncovering Intergenerational Cycles of Violence

Kenneth X. Robbins, M.D.

The story of King Oedipus of Thebes plays a central role in the history of psychoanalysis. Freud based his theory of the Oedipus complex on the "Greek myth of King Oedipus, whose destiny it was to slay his father and to wed his mother, who did all in his power to avoid the fate prophesied by the oracle, and who in self-punishment blinded himself when he discovered that in ignorance he had committed both these crimes" (Freud 1935, p. 290). In 1897, he wrote to Fliess that "I have found love of the mother and jealousy of the father in my own case too, and now believe it to be a general phenomenon of early childhood. . . . The Greek myth seizes on a compulsion which everyone recognizes because he has felt traces of it in himself" (Freud 1954, pp. 223–224). Psychoanalytic theorists have considered oedipal themes universal because generational competition and incest prohibition are thought to be a basis for human interactions in all societies.

The myth cycle relating to Oedipus and other members of the royal family of Thebes describes a world fraught with intergenerational and intragenerational conflict and violence. In addition to tales of patricide and incest, there are accounts of many crimes and breaches of taboos, including infanticide, abandonment and killing of children, fratricide, and out-of-wedlock pregnancy. Only by retelling the entire family history can the case of Oedipus be put into perspective as part of a pattern of continuing multigenerational familial dysfunction in a

The author thanks Lowell Edmunds, Professor of Classics at Rutgers University, for his critique and review of this chapter.

violent lineage noted for breaching norms, biological as well as societal. According to Marcel Detienne, "What . . . created mythology was the sense of the scandalous in myth. Myth was the Other of religion, reason, or civilization. Mythology rose to explain scandal" (Edmunds 1990, p. 1).

The royal family of Thebes was a favorite subject of Greek myth, epic, and tragic drama. Many important epics and plays about their lives and exploits have been lost. There is no guarantee that surviving versions were the most important or definitive ones in ancient times. The *Thebaid* and *Oedipodeia,* two epics similar in scope to the *Iliad* and the *Odyssey,* are known only from fragmentary references. What if lost Greek tragedies such as Thespis' *Pentheus,* Aeschylus' *Laius,* and Euripides' *Oedipus* had survived? Some "facts" central to many modern interpretations turn out to be variants in conflict with accounts in other ancient versions. For example, in some ancient accounts, Oedipus did not blind himself, and he continued to rule in Thebes until his death in battle.

If the entire myth cycle is recounted, readers might be overwhelmed by the large number of unfamiliar names and confusing episodes. Therefore, some psychological interpreters select only one element or variant that buttresses their own theories. The clarity and consistency of such studies are achieved at the cost of ignoring most of the data. Only a full retelling can reveal repetitive thematic patterns within the myth cycle.

Data whose meaning is obscure or anxiety-provoking should not be ignored or discarded. In myth as sometimes in life, contradictions are not resolved but are stressed and exaggerated as conflicting stories are incorporated into the circulating corpus. In this way, myth deals with the fundamental contradictions inherent in life. Inconsistencies and variations should be compared because they may reveal conflictual situations and controversial material, otherwise hidden. Edmunds (1990) describes the origin and importance of variants:

> Each retelling or application produces a new variant, which stands in some degree of antagonistic relationship to other variants or other myths and thus takes its place in a system constituted by the proliferation of such relations. . . . Myths are never neutral but always have some point in the context in which they are told, and thus in principle they demand an answer. (pp. 4, 15)

The Royal Family of Thebes (Figure 1–1)

Agenor was unable to protect his daughter Europa from the attentions of the god Zeus, who, taking the form of a bull, kidnapped and ravished her. Agenor told Cadmus and his other sons to find her or never return home. Cadmus's mother left her husband to journey with Cadmus. After her death, the Delphic oracle told Cadmus to terminate his search for Europa (and the bull) and settle where a specially marked cow would rest.

Founding a city on the spot where the cow rested was not easy. Several of Cadmus's men were slain by a dragon guarding a spring sacred to the god Ares. Therefore, Cadmus slew the beast. His patron goddess Athena told him to sow the dragon's teeth in the ground. Each tooth immediately turned into a warrior who tried to kill the others. All fell except Echion, Chthonius, and three other Sown-men or Spartoi, who became the progenitors of the new settlement. Cadmus served Ares to atone for killing the dragon and was granted the hand of the god's daughter Harmonia. Despite this marital alliance, Ares continued to punish his son-in-law Cadmus by inflicting disasters on his own grandchildren and even their descendants. In the end, Ares transformed Cadmus and Harmonia into snakes, either as a punishment or as a sign of perpetual honor.

Cadmus's daughter Semele had an illegitimate son, Dionysus. According to the tradition of the coastal town of Brasiae, Cadmus threw them into the sea in a trunk. The most popular version claims that Dionysus had more than two parents. First Zeus in the form of a snake lay with Persephone. His jealous wife Hera had the Titans eat the child, but Zeus managed to swallow the heart. He impregnated Semele by giving her the heart to drink. Hera (or Semele's jealous sister Ino) tricked Semele into demanding that Zeus appear to her in his true form. When he did, she was consumed by lightning. Once again, Zeus rescued the unborn child by sewing him into his thigh.

Semele's sister Ino and her husband Athamas were punished by Hera with madness for protecting their nephew Dionysus. The madness took the form of trying to kill their own children. Athamas, mistaking his son Learchus for a deer or lion cub, shot him with an arrow. Ino boiled their other son Melicertes or jumped into the sea with him. Ino also tried to kill Athamas's children by his first wife Nephele. Ino persuaded the women to tamper with the city's seed and bribed messen-

Figure 1–1. *(At right)* Genealogical chart of the Royal House of Thebes, the family of Oedipus.

Key
Males—Names written in capital letters.
Females—Names written in upper and lowercase letters.
Deities—Names underlined.
Kings of Thebes—Names written in capital letters on black background.

1. Dionysus had two mothers and was called the "Twice-born" (see text).
2. The paternity of Antiope's children was disputed (see text).
3. Jocasta was the wife of Oedipus as well as his mother.
4. Information was not available to indicate the order of birth.

gers from the Oracle at Delphi to say that her stepson Phrixus must be sacrificed to avoid famine. Phrixus was miraculously saved while his father Athamas was attempting to sacrifice him. Like Isaac, Phrixus was rescued by the sudden appearance of another sacrifice in the form of a ram. Other variants have Nephele saving Phrixus and her daughter Helle by having them escape on the back of a flying ram with golden fleece.

Learchus was not the only one of Cadmus's grandsons to be slain by intimates who mistook him for a beast. The great hunter Actaeon accidentally viewed the goddess Artemis in her bath and was punished by being torn apart by his own hounds who mistook him for a stag. Some explanations claim that Actaeon's crime was that he wished to marry his aunt Semele. King Pentheus was torn apart by his mother Agave and aunts who were in the midst of rites in honor of Dionysus, who had recently returned to the city.

Even Cadmus recognized the divine nature of his grandson Dionysus, whom he had previously cast into the sea as a bastard. The blind seer Teiresias, a priest of Apollo, left his normal state of sobriety to join the ecstatic rites. Pentheus alone failed to recognize Dionysus's status. The outraged god cast a spell transforming the behavior of his puritanical, overcontrolled, and hypermasculine cousin into that of a female bacchant. Dressed in female garb, Pentheus broke the taboo against males viewing the Bacchic orgies and reveled in thoughts of being held by his mother. His mother Agave did not recognize him, leading him to plaintively cry out like a frightened child: "It is I, mother, your son Pentheus." Despite this, the women, led by Agave,

THE ROYAL HOUSE OF THEBES

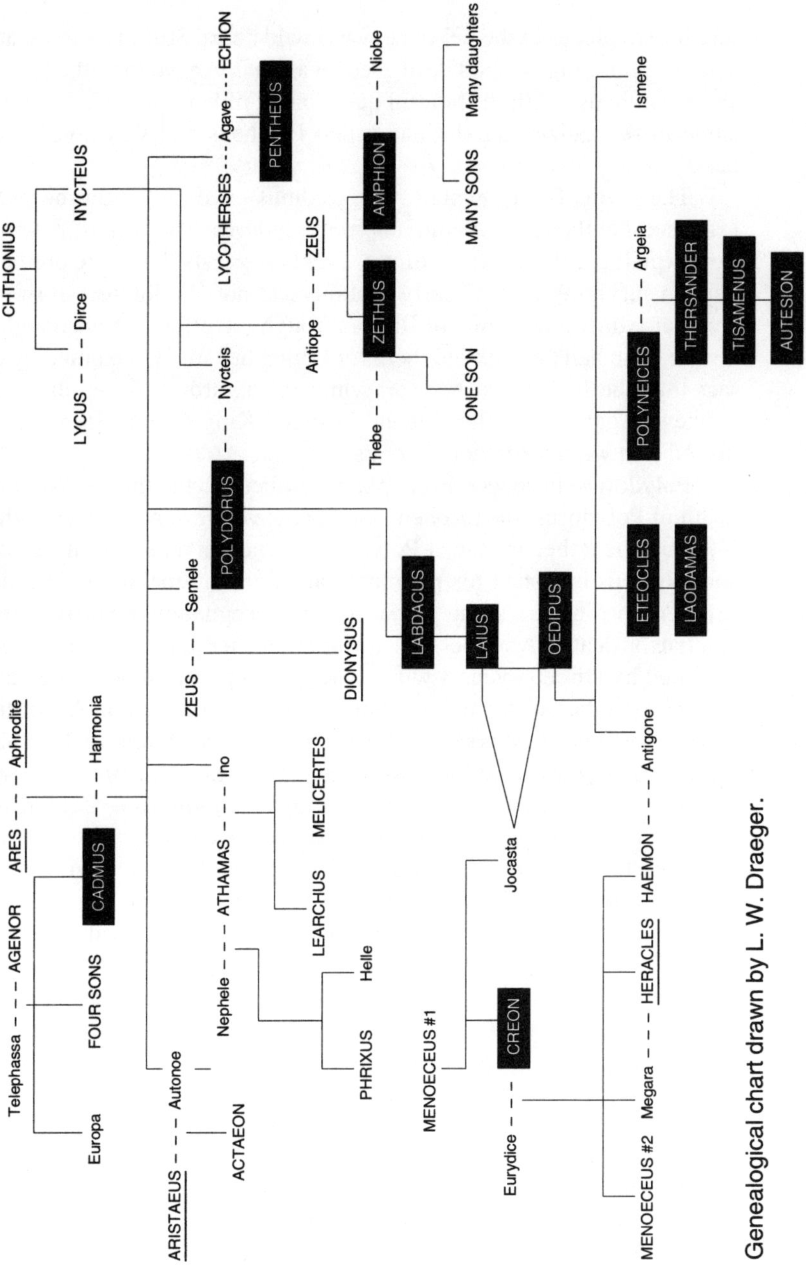

Genealogical chart drawn by L. W. Draeger.

tore him to pieces in the belief he was a wild beast. Still in a dissociated state and thinking she had destroyed an animal, Agave took the head to show Pentheus. With the helpful questioning of her father Cadmus, she came to recognize that she had killed Pentheus and was holding his head.

The myths fail to explain why Cadmus gave up his throne to his grandson Pentheus, bypassing his son Polydorus. The lack of information explaining these extraordinary events suggests that there are large gaps in surviving data. Clearly Cadmus had not lost interest in ruling. He later gained the throne of Illyria through the efforts of his daughter Agave, who had been exiled there for killing her son. Undaunted by the fact that she had killed her son while in rapturous adoration of her nephew, Agave killed her second husband King Lycotherses and replaced him with her father Cadmus.

Polydorus succeeded his nephew Pentheus to the throne. After the death of Polydorus, the throne passed to his young son Labdacus while Nycteus, the father-in-law of Polydorus, served as regent for his grandson. Nycteus banished his pregnant daughter Antiope and killed himself. According to some versions, the pregnancy occurred after Nycteus's death. Antiope was tortured by her uncle Lycus or imprisoned by Dirce (Lycus's wife). The god Zeus was among the many different candidates for the paternity of Antiope's children. According to some versions, Lycus seduced Antiope. In others, Lycus and Antiope were married, but the children were fathered by the King of Sicyon who impersonated Lycus. In any case, Antiope's twin sons Zethus and Amphion were abandoned and exposed to die by Lycus.

Like his first cousin Pentheus, King Labdacus was literally torn apart by female worshipers of his cousin Dionysus. This may suggest strong intragenerational rivalries for power within the royal family; or it may be that Labdacus was maturing and wanted to wield the reins of power. In any case, Lycus was able to retain power as regent under Labdacus's infant son Laius. Soon the twins Amphion and Zethus, who survived exposure, seized power from Laius and Lycus.

The citadel continued to be named Cadmeia after Cadmus until, for unknown reasons, the metropolis was renamed Thebes in honor of Thebe, Zethus's wife. Thebe never really held any power. She tried to kill the children of Niobe, her sister-in-law. Instead, she mistakenly slew her own son and was transformed into a nightingale. In the end, the children of the prideful Niobe were slain not by Thebe but by

Apollo and Artemis, angered because Niobe boasted that she had more children than the mother of these gods.

Meanwhile, Laius sought sanctuary with Pelops, a brother-in-law of his enemy Amphion. Laius is said to have abused Pelops's hospitality by kidnapping and seducing his host's son Chrysippus who in some versions later committed suicide. Another version claims that Laius and his son Oedipus fought over the favors of Chrysippus, something that could only have occurred much later in Laius's life.

Alternate versions claim that Chrysippus was murdered by his half-brothers Atreus and Thyestes, whose mother feared Chrysippus would succeed to the throne. Naturally, throwing the blame on Laius, an outsider, would help maintain family solidarity if this was the nature of the crime. Pelops, said to have cursed Laius for acts against Chrysippus, had already been cursed himself for killing someone. Pelops killed Oenomaus so he could marry his daughter; an oracle warned him that he would die at the hands of his daughter's husband. Pelops's descendants continued the family tradition of betrayal and violence, which included adultery, child neglect and rejection, child sacrifice and killing, matricide, spousal murder, and cannibalism. The myth cycle of Pelops's family terminates with the story of Orestes who does not commit incest with his mother but kills her to avenge the murder of his father. Following the deaths of Amphion and Zethus, Laius returned to Thebes and regained the throne. He married Jocasta, who was descended from one of the Spartoi. The Oracle at Delphi told him that if he had a son, the child would kill him. The tragedies that were to befall him and his family were said to be related to his breach of Pelops's hospitality or the oracle's instructions not to impregnate his wife. Laius may have had his own reasons to avoid heterosexual intercourse; the ancients considered him the founder of pederasty.

Laius avoided sex until Jocasta succeeded in getting him intoxicated so she could seduce him. The product of that union was a son who was rejected. According to some versions, he was cast into the sea in a chest and found by the Queen of Corinth. Other ancient writers wrote that he was exposed to die on a mountain. Accounts often state that a spike was driven through the child's feet, suggesting that the child could already walk when he was exposed. Like Dionysus and the twins Amphion and Zethus, he survived the experience of being thrown away by members of his family. A shepherd gave him to King Polybus and Queen Periboea (also known as Merope) of Corinth, who raised him as their own son. The child was named Oedipus, which means "Swollen Foot" or possibly "Son of the Swelling Sea," referring to the different stories of his exposure.

Oedipus was startled when told that Polybus and Periboea were not his parents. Apparently, he had not been told of his true origins and went to the oracle for information. She drove him away, stating he would kill his father and marry his mother.

Oedipus did not return to Corinth or reflect on his true parentage. Certainly, he must have been familiar with fosterage, the Greek custom of raising aristocratic children at a different court or with another family (Bremmer 1988). Still angry and confused, he encountered an overbearing man who belligerently demanded that Oedipus let him pass first at a triple crossroads. (A triple crossroads was a site haunted by the terrible underworld goddess Hecate as well as the place where Plato advocated the stoning of patricides.) In the ensuing fight, Oedipus killed this man, though the stranger was old enough to be his father. In fact, this man was Laius.

Oedipus came to Thebes where the Sphinx, a winged female monster with a woman's head and a lion's body, was eating men who were unable to answer a riddle: "What is it that goes on four legs in the morning, two during the day, and three at night?" or in the fuller version of Athenaeus "There walks on land a creature of two feet, of four feet, and of three feet; it has but one voice, but sole among animals that grow on land or in the sea, it can change its nature; nay, when it walks propped on most feet, then is the speed of its limbs less than it has ever been before" (Bremmer 1988; Edmunds 1985). The throne and the hand of Jocasta were offered to the man who could defeat the Sphinx. Oedipus answered "Man." The Sphinx then destroyed herself.

Who was the Sphinx? According to Pausanius, the Sphinx was a brigand who sought the throne as the illegitimate daughter of Laius. According to most accounts, she was a winged composite monster. She was a daughter of Echidna, who was half-snake and half-nymph, and hundred-snakeheaded Typhaon or their two-dogheaded son Orthus. In other words, like the children of Oedipus, the Sphinx may have been conceived as a result of mother-son incest.

Oedipus became King of Thebes, apparently continuing a system whereby the throne was gained by marrying the queen of the last monarch. Of course, this conflicts with all the data about succession given previously. Some scholars have claimed that Oedipus tried to substitute patrilineal for matrilineal laws of succession (Graves 1955, p. 15). To satisfy both sets of rules, the previous king would have been considered his father and the queen the consort first of the father and then of the son.

Oedipus begot two sons, Eteocles and Polyneices, and two daughters, Antigone and Ismene. According to Pherecydes, there were two additional sons, Phrastor and Laonytus, neither mentioned elsewhere. Though some versions state that a wife named Euryganeia was the mother of Oedipus's children, it is usually said that the children's mother was Jocasta, the wife of Oedipus and (unbeknownst to him) his mother.

Oedipus saw himself as a self-made man, never realizing that he was born to become King of Thebes. In his own eyes, he had escaped the horrible fate forecast for him. He saw himself as omniscient and invulnerable.

After many prosperous years, a plague devastated Thebes because the murderer of Laius had not been punished. Oedipus condemned the unknown murderer to severe punishment. Oedipus forced Teiresias to name the murderer. When told he himself was the criminal, he became irate accusing his brother-in-law Creon and the seer of plotting against him. Eventually, the truth of the prophet's statements was confirmed. Oedipus had fulfilled the oracle's prediction that he would commit patricide and marry his mother. According to Sophocles, Jocasta hanged herself and Oedipus blinded himself with her brooches. (According to Apollodorus and Euripides, the ankles of the young Oedipus had been pierced with brooches before he was exposed.) According to Seneca, Jocasta thrust Oedipus's sword into her "capacious womb." Jocasta, like the Sphinx, killed herself after Oedipus solved a puzzle. Some versions state that Oedipus tore his eyes from his own sockets. Following this fall from high position and prestige, Oedipus became an exiled outcast. He became a blind, helpless beggar, the very names he had flung in rage at Teiresias.

A number of ancient sources including the *Iliad* give a markedly different account of the later life of Oedipus, saying that he was neither blinded nor exiled but continued to rule Thebes until his death, possibly in battle against the Minyans of Orkhomenos. According to Hesiod, he was honored at his death with funeral games. In Euripides' *Phoenician Women,* Jocasta kills herself years later and then only over the dead bodies of her sons by Oedipus.

Oedipus did not treat his sons well. According to the *Thebaid,* he cursed them because they served him with the Theban royal cups of his father, which he had forbidden, and fed him with an inferior cut of meat from a sacrificial animal.

Eteocles and Polyneices did nothing to help Oedipus. Euripides wrote that they imprisoned him in a dark place, hoping to dissociate themselves from his polluting acts. Eteocles and his uncle Creon wanted to bury him alive outside the walls of Thebes so that his cursed tomb could protect Thebes against invasion.

Oedipus wandered for years, accursed and accompanied by Antigone, his daughter-sister who cared for him like a mother. His sons and Creon sought his return to Thebes, but not out of concern for him. They knew of the auspiciousness to be associated with the site of his tomb. Oedipus continued to curse them, making no attempt to reconcile with them.

Theseus, king of Athens, protected him against Creon, Eteocles, and Polyneices. Theseus, like Oedipus, had been sent to certain death by his father, had slain a composite monster, was unwittingly responsible for his father's death, was banished at the end of his reign, and was part of an oedipal triangle. (Theseus's wife Phaedra tried to seduce his son Hippolytus into stepmother-stepson "incest.")

Oedipus entered a grove at Colonus dedicated to the Eumenides, awesome goddesses who ensured the fertility of the earth. Aeschylus identified them with the Erinyes, female spirits who punished matricide and other crimes against blood kin. Such suprahuman retribution was deemed necessary to uphold the hierarchical principle of obedience and respect for parents. Oedipus did not suffer punishment for entering the sacred precincts. Once again, he had committed a forbidden act, but this time he was redeemed in the process.

Oedipus had committed acts like patricide and mother-son incest that were ritually polluting. Though he admitted these polluting acts, Oedipus insisted that he never *knowingly* did anything wrong. He asks "when I am nothing—then am I a man?" His daughter Ismene told him that the gods, once bent on his destruction, now will "raise you to your feet." Oedipus replied that "it costs them little to raise an old man, someone crushed in younger days." His prideful boasts that he controlled his own destiny and his pretensions to omniscience were no longer heard. Oedipus recognized the nature of human limitations. He became "the mediator between chthonic and Olympian powers and stands in a privileged relation to the goddesses who embody both the destructive and creative forces of nature" (Segal 1986, p. 31). The site of the tomb of Oedipus was kept secret, bringing good fortune to Athens as well as protecting the city against Theban aggression.

Oedipus never reconciled with the males in his family lineage. As he predicted, his sons were unable to lovingly divide their inheritance. They shared the throne until Eteocles banished his brother.

Polyneices, aided by his father-in-law King Adrastus of Argos, attacked Thebes. Teiresias told Creon that, in order to save Thebes, his son Menoeceus must be sacrificed to Ares. Disregarding Creon's admonition to flee, Menoeceus killed himself in the cave where Cadmus slew Ares's dragon.

In battle, Polyneices and Eteocles slew each other. Antigone gave her brother Polyneices the funeral rites forbidden by Creon because he had attacked the city. She committed suicide as did her fiance Haemon, who was Creon's son. In a lost play, *Antigone,* Euripides had Haemon impregnate Antigone and arrange for shepherds to smuggle her away. Their son later came to Thebes and was recognized by Creon through a birthmark common to all descendants of the Spartoi. Unable to move his angry father, Haemon killed Antigone and himself.

Laodamas, the son of Eteocles, was placed on the throne with Creon as regent. Lycus, a descendent of Lycus previously described, killed Creon, usurping the throne. He was killed by Creon's son-in-law Heracles, and Laodamas was restored to the throne. Thebes was seized by the Epigoni, sons of the Argive warriors who had attacked the city under Polyneices. The latter's son Thersander became king and died in the Trojan War. Little is recorded of the rule of his son Tisamenus, but his grandson Autesion was forced to give up the throne. He was so hounded by the ghosts of his ancestors Laius and Oedipus that, following oracular advice, he left Thebes forever. Thus, the story of Oedipus ends not with crimes by a son against his parents but by another in a long series of hostilities by ancestors, parents, older relatives, siblings, and cousins against the younger members of the Theban royal family!

Oedipus Myths and Hostility Toward Children

The Theban attitude toward children is one of fear and animosity. No child is safe from the anger of caretakers, strangers, and parents or the hostility of mortals and immortals. Agave, Thebe, Athamas, and Ino kill their sons. Lycus usurps the throne of Laius, tortures his niece

Antiope, and exposes her twin sons. Laius exposes his son Oedipus, who later curses his own sons. Even death does not still wrath against descendants as the shades (ghosts) of Laius and Oedipus haunt the last of their royal descendants.

Over and over, parents deny hostile intentions against the children they attack. Repeatedly, they claim that they did not recognize their children because some deity clouded their vision or they were attempting to enhance the child's position (in some cases by removing potential rivals). There is no information given suggesting that any male figure in the royal house of Thebes had a supportive relationship with his father.

Repeatedly, Theban children are punished for the misdeeds of parents. Ares persecuted generations of Thebans (though they were the progeny of his daughter) because Cadmus killed his sacred dragon. Even innocent children are punished. For example, Ares demands the sacrifice of Creon's son Menoeceus because Menoeceus is an innocent virgin.

Though acts against infant and young males are repeatedly described, female infanticide is not mentioned at all. Women are discussed only in terms of their relationship with men. The sexual behavior or experiences of Semele and Antiope represented threats to family honor or stability and therefore are mentioned. There is a warning given in stories of heavy penalties suffered by Actaeon, Pentheus, and Teiresias for breaching the taboo against viewing women that "did not belong" to them. Yet there is no mention of father-daughter incest, probably because this represented little threat to the hierarchical, patriarchal society portrayed in this myth cycle.

Women are torn between their obligations to their families of origin, their husbands, and their sons. Agave favors her nephew over her son and her father over her second husband; this results in the murders of Pentheus and Lycotherses. Antigone gives up any chance for a happy life with Haemon when she defies her uncle (and soon to be father-in-law) by burying her brother. Ino and Thebe try to kill young males whose claims might rival those of their own sons.

Oedipus Myths and Disorders of Narcissism

This myth cycle deals with the question of the limits of human behavior and the consequences of hubris (excess pride). Humans may seek knowledge and power by breaching taboos. Very often such acts lead to an outcome contrary to a person's avowed intentions. Ino and Thebe murder their own children while attempting to murder their sons' potential rivals. Oedipus takes the precise course of action ensuring fulfillment of the prophecy whose consequences he seeks to avoid. Eventually this leads to a dramatic recognition of the limitations of human power and ability to control one's own destiny.

The societal consequences of certain proscribed acts are complex. Punishment and suffering of the perpetrator can occur even if the act was not knowingly and freely committed. In such a case, the person is responsible though not technically guilty. Succeeding generations may bear the brunt of a forebear's deeds. According to the Greeks, the negative effects of such acts may affect society in general—as in the case of Thebes, which was ravaged by a plague because the murderer of Laius had gone unpunished.

The position of one who is so impure as to pollute all of society is such that his presence may also be auspicious. In the case of Oedipus, his presence pollutes the entire city, but his tomb would protect it. Such is the link of Oedipus to patterns of sacral kingship: "In Tragedy . . . the king occupies the symbolic point where the human and the divine intersect. His sufferings represent the efforts of the society to maintain those relations with the cosmic order on which its physical and spiritual life depends" (Segal 1986, p. 29).

Some people try to transcend societal and personal limitations by breaching taboos (in fact or fantasy), such as the prohibition against incest or murder. In this way, like Oedipus, they can become true members of the royal house of Thebes, achieving what Aristotle considered an ambiguous status outside of human society as either monster or god. The therapist must consider the possibility that such behavior and fantasy, however heinous or "impure," may result in a sense of being special or auspicious or achieving that status in the eyes of others.

A feeling of being "special" may result from interaction with an overly close or incestuous parent. The intense conflict between this feeling and all the negative feelings may overwhelm a young psyche. Even as an adult, the victim may not be able to detach from such an interaction, however debasing and degrading. Some victims consider physical abuse evidence of concern and will say "he only hits me because he cares." Humiliation is equated with love. Incest victims may feel soiled and "polluted." A woman who was forcibly abused as a child came to therapy because she had the feeling that "nothing can ever go right for anyone if I am involved. I am and always will be a cesspool of pollution."

The omniscient-omnipotent person, such as Oedipus, sees himself as a self-made man. Having solved some great problem, he assumes that this action will carry him through life. Like Oedipus, his answer to the riddle of life is to hide emotional deprivation and/or abuse behind a facade proclaiming that he can and must be successful by his own efforts. The following is a clinical example.

> An intermittently depressed man considered himself successful. His mother died when he was young. When he was 16, his father killed himself, and he was cast out by his stepmother. Despite this, he was successful in the military and attained high rank. His marriage was cold and loveless. His daughter was isolated; his nonfunctioning son killed himself. The man voiced great sadness over these tragedies; yet even after his retirement, his efforts remained focused on his professional interests, not family matters. In group therapy, he told a man who had unexpectedly and suddenly heard voices: "It's okay as long as you can go to work."

The Theban myth cycle repeatedly deals with the theme that excesses lead to hubris, the "sin" of pride and arrogance. Niobe arrogantly boasted about the number of her children, and the blindly prideful Oedipus insisted he could and would solve any mystery or riddle. Both were humiliated to teach us the importance of humility.

The belief that humiliation brings humility and prevents hubris tends to be a recurrent theme in the lives of masochistic or self-defeating people.

> A woman repeatedly snatched defeat out of the jaws of victory. Whenever she achieved any goal, she felt uncertain, uncomfortable, and needed to undo the "victory" by cutting herself or creating chaos in some other area of her life. She developed an intense rivalry with another patient in group who also basked in his self-defeating behavior and called himself "The King of Pain Mountain." Her ambition was to be like "The Anchorman," the student finishing dead last in academic standing at the Naval Academy. "The Anchorman" has a special auspicious status; to know him or her is considered lucky.

The Clinical Importance of Mythical Thinking by the Therapist

The term mythical thinking means a particular way of organizing experience and perceiving the self. Each person, every family, and all cultures have an ongoing need to shape and reshape the special myths that guide conduct, describe goals, assign blame, and create a cohesive view of life and self. Without such dynamic myths, both the sense of self and the perception of the world would seem amorphous and troubling. The world is a place where dichotomous categories may collapse or blur and where different sets of such categories may be in conflict.

In the myth cycle retold previously, there is confusion and ambiguity in classification, hierarchical differentiation (e.g., in the case of Jocasta, who is both mother and wife to Oedipus), social obligations (e.g., Antigone's conflict between the need to bury a dead relative and the political prohibition against such an act) and even the linguistic code (replete with riddles, cryptic oracles, and even a chief character whose name has several meanings). Such problems are inherent in human thought and experience. There is a constant struggle to understand and orient oneself in relation to both self and the world.

No psychotherapist can hope to grasp immediately all the nuances of any individual's life history and psychiatric problems. Though interventions and tentative formulations must be made on an ongoing basis, therapists should resist the urge to restrict data selection and interpretation in a reductionistic manner for the sake of "clarity." In any ongoing therapy, unclear or confusing information should not be discarded, because its import may only come clear as more information or patterns emerge. For example, the meanings of a single dream may only become clear in comparison to other dreams.

Confusion and contradiction should be accepted as inevitable in explanations of conflictual or traumatic situations.

> A woman recalling her poor relationship with her mother revealed that "a lot that has come down to me through gossip, surmise on my part, and Mama's biased tales that kept changing through the years. I still don't know which versions are true, which are base lies, and which are wishful thinking on Mama's part."

Contradictions may actually define the nature of the clinical problem, as in the case of the double bind where a person is asked to perform two mutually exclusive acts and cannot get clarification as to which takes precedence.

Transparently erroneous or contradictory statements made by seemingly nondelusional persons may seem unshakable.

> For example, a woman told the therapist that her daughter had contracted gonorrhea from a toilet seat when she was 11. (At that time, the girl was sharing a bedroom with her grandfather.) Despite the fact that she was a registered nurse, the woman vehemently insisted that her daughter's case was the one exception to the rule that gonorrhea could not be contracted from toilet seats.

This illustrates a point repeatedly made in the myth cycle: When family solidarity or honor is threatened by something, such as an illegitimate pregnancy, this must be explained away by recourse to tales of exceptional circumstances, such as liaisons with gods. Even when misdeeds are acknowledged, responsibility may be denied. For example, in the myth cycle, Agave and Ino attributed the slaying of their own children to the malevolent powers of the gods, not their own desires. However, they also cold-bloodedly tried to murder other family members, suggesting that they might also have had murderous feelings toward the sons they slaughtered.

Often, patients are unaware of how family myths arise to cover or excuse hostile or negative feelings.

> An elderly woman and her son claimed that their family had always insisted on absolute individual freedom of choice and that, therefore, no one had the right to control or influence another family member. She and her son took it as a matter of family pride and honor that this principle was never breached, even when her depressed suicidal husband purchased a gun for the explicit purpose of killing himself. (She even left the house knowing he would then shoot himself.) Yet it was untrue that the principle had never been breached: Years before, the entire family had confronted the woman's husband about his alcoholism, resulting in his 12 years of sobriety. The woman considered his suicide "the greatest gift he ever gave me."

Personal and family myths are not static but are dynamic and interactive. Each story is retold and reinterpreted in light of new experiences and further psychological development. To produce an appropriate synthesis, the dominant myth needs to take into account its antithesis with "reciprocal assimilation and accommodations" between them (Feinstein et al. 1988, p. 34). It is pragmatic in taking patient and family histories to record all contradictions, omissions, and emphases, as these reflect information about both the informant and the family. In effect, each version represents a selection of data that is then shaped into a coherent story reflecting the experience and personality of the informant. Such selection is the end product of the repression of unconscious conflicts as well as dissociation of aggressive and sexual traumas. The missing material may be found or explained in other versions of the same stories or similar ones. Therefore, psychiatric evaluation should include a genealogical history and longitudinal life history and, when practical, information from family members and past therapists.

Genealogical information often reveals similarities in the world outlook and problem areas of family members over several generations.

> A woman with multiple personality disorder had many symptoms similar to those of her mother, as well as some that seemed to have recurred over a number of generations, from a distant ancestor to a cousin 20 years her junior. This became evident only when the cousin located her, seeking genealogical information to help her understand her own problems. There was a familial pattern of sexual and physical abuse and degradation of children as well as many breaches of conventional standards. Both the woman and her mother had been abused as children; both had abused their own children.

If enough major elements of the story are suppressed, repressed, dissociated, or discarded in a reductionistic manner, coherence and clarity may be attained at the cost of psychic and objective reality.

> A depressed man announced that he thought he had been "immunized" against mental illness by the fact that his father was a world-famous psychologist specializing in child development. He failed to mention that his alcoholic father was chronically depressed as well as withdrawn and nonfunctional and that he himself had never been "psychologically minded."

The need to present a situation as a coherent organic unity may result in a formulation reflecting the views of the formulator as well as the situation. The Theban plays of Sophocles emphasize the misdeeds of sons, not fathers; this may reflect Sophocles's acrimonious battles with his own son Iophon. The formulations and theories of therapists may reflect a need to decrease their own cognitive dissonance as well as intolerance for ambiguity and uncomfortable affects. It is always tempting to pigeonhole and categorize in a familiar though reductionistic manner rather than deal with the unfamiliar, atypical, or confusing situations. In such situations, the pejorative use of the labels like "borderline" can be used inappropriately to eliminate the need to understand a person in depth. Interpretations should not be limited to those most easily accommodated to the therapist's theoretical orientation. Most psychoanalytic articles consider the Sphinx only as a maternal figure; the many alternate explanations clearly given in the myths themselves are rarely even mentioned. Similarly, a patient's interpretations are important even if they are obscure or seem different than those accepted by the therapist. If a patient senses that the therapist has difficulty dealing with any issue, the patient may withhold information.

Some patients come to therapy with the expectation that the therapist is an oracle who can answer all their questions. Such people may be dismayed when subjected to questions or when their requests for advice are not directly answered. The Oracle at Delphi had advice written on the wall urging the individual asking for information to "Know yourself." The cryptic responses of the oracle seem to have been based in the concept that self-examination will reveal that the questions asked reflect one's own unconscious desires and fears and one's dissociated traumatic experiences.

Essential to an empathic therapeutic relationship is the therapist's ability to tolerate uncertainty as well as the therapist's ability to validate the feelings of others without necessarily agreeing with them completely. Uncertainty and conflicting desires are to be expected and can be seen as the part of human development allowing for diversity, complexity, and change by a dialectical process incorporating all alternatives and opposites. Such mythical thinking by the therapist serves as a counterbalance and check against reductionism based on the therapist's personal anxieties, blind spots, etiological assumptions, and cultural beliefs.

References

Bremmer J: Oedipus and the Greek Oedipus complex, in Interpretations of Greek Mythology. Edited by Bremmer J. London, Routledge, 1988

Edmunds L: Oedipus: The Ancient Legend and Its Later Analogues. Baltimore, MD, Johns Hopkins University Press, 1985

Feinstein D, Krippner S, Granger D: Mythmaking and human development. Journal of Humanistic Psychology 28(3):23–50, 1988

Graves R: The Greek Myths, Vol Two. Baltimore, MD, Penguin, 1955

Segal C: Interpreting Greek Tragedy: Myth, Poetry, Text. Ithaca, NY, Cornell University Press, 1986

Suggested Readings

Caldwell RS: The Blindness of Oedipus. International Review of Psycho-Analysis 1:207–218, 1974

Caldwell R: The psychoanalytic interpretation of Greek myth, in Approaches to Greek Myth. Edited by Edmunds L. Baltimore, MD, Johns Hopkins University Press, 1990, pp 344–389

Carroll MP: Levi-Strauss on the Oedipus myth: a reconsideration. American Anthropologist 80:805–814, 1978

Datan N: After Oedipus: Laius, Medea, and other parental myths. Journal of Mind and Behavior 3:17–26, 1982

Datan N: The Oedipus cycle: developmental mythology, Greek tragedy, and the sociology of knowledge. Int J Aging Hum Dev 27:1–10, 1988

D'Aulaire I, D'Aulaire E: D'Aulaire's Book of Greek Myths. Garden City, NY, Doubleday, 1962

Devereux G: The psychotherapy scene in Euripides' Bacchae. Journal of Hellenic Studies 90:35–48, 1970

Dodds E: On misunderstanding the Oedipus Rex. Greece and Rome 13:37–49, 1966

Edmunds L: Freud and the father: Oedipus Complex and Oedipus myth. Psychoanalysis and Contemporary Thought 8:87–103, 1985

Edmunds L: The practice of Greek mythology, in Approaches to Greek Myth. Edited by Edmunds L. Baltimore, MD, Johns Hopkins University Press, 1990, pp 1–20

Freud S: A General Introduction to Psychoanalysis. New York, Liveright Publishing, 1935

Freud S: The Origins of Psychoanalysis: Letters to Wilhelm Fliess, Notes and Drafts. New York, Basic Books, 1954

Fromm E: The Oedipus Complex and the Oedipus Myth in The Family: Its Function and Destiny. Edited by Anshen R. New York, Harper & Row, 1948, pp 420–448

Goleman D: Personal myths bring cohesion to the chaos of each life. New York Times, May 24, 1988, pp C1, C11

Grant M: Myths of the Greeks and the Romans. New York, Mentor, 1962

Graves R: The Greek Myths: I. Hammondsworth, Middlesex, England, Penguin, 1960

Kamerbeck J: The Plays of Sophocles. Commentaries Part IV: The Oedipus Tyrannus. Leiden, Netherlands, Brill EJ, 1967

Knox B: Sophocles' Oedipus, in Tragic Themes in Western Literature. Edited by Brooks C. New Haven, CT, Yale University Press, 1955, pp 7–29

Levi-Strauss C: The structural theory of myth, in Myth: A Symposium. Edited by Sebeok T. Bloomington, IN, Indiana University Press, 1955, pp 81–106

Lidz T: The Riddle of the Riddle of the Sphinx. Psychoanal Rev 75:35–49, 1988

O'Brien MJ: Twentieth Century Interpretations of Oedipus Rex. Edited by O'Brien MJ. Englewood Cliffs, NJ, Prentice-Hall, 1968

Reinhold M: Classical Drama: Greek and Roman. Great Neck, NY, Barron's Educational Series, 1959

Robbins KX: The World of Oedipus. Paper presented at the Washington School of Psychiatry Conference, "The Kingdom of Oedipus," June 1988

Robbins KX: Oedipal themes in Hindu mythology, art, history and culture. Paper presented at Columbia University Southeast Asian Institute, September 1992

Ross JM: Oedipus revisited: Laius and the Laius complex. Psychoanal Study Child 37:169–200, 1982

Rudnytsky PL: Freud and Oedipus. New York, Columbia University Press, 1987

Schavrien JE: The rage, healing and daemonic death of Oedipus: a self-in-relation theory. Journal of Transpersonal Psychology 21:149–176, 1989

Sophocles: The Three Theban Plays. New York, Penguin, 1982

Taylor DC: Oedipus' parents were child abusers. Br J Psychiatry 153:561–563, 1988

Tripp E: The Meridian Handbook of Classical Mythology. New York, Meridian, 1970

Willner D: The Oedipus Complex, Antigone, and Electra: the woman as hero and victim. American Anthropologist 84:58–78, 1982

Chapter 2

Electra: Revenge Fantasies and Homicide in Child Abuse Victims

Jeffrey Richards, M.D.
Jean M. Goodwin, M.D., M.P.H.

Introduction

The Electra Complex is usually thought of as the female version of the Oedipus Complex: the little girl imagines herself killing mother and marrying father (Jung 1961). However, while Electra did connive in the murder of her mother, Clytemnestra, she, unlike Oedipus, was in no position to marry the opposite sex parent (her father, Agamemnon); he had been killed long before by Electra's mother. In fact, Agamemnon's murder was only one in a series of acts of family violence. These included the intrafamilial killings of at least five of Electra's siblings or half-siblings and the attempted murder of her brother; one half-sister killed herself.

Many theorists have felt the concept of the Electra Complex needs revision, including Freud, who wrote about Jung's 1913 conceptualization: "I do not see any advance or gain in the introduction of the term 'Electra Complex' and do not advocate its use" (Freud 1920/1955, p. 155).

In our discussion here, Electra's obsessions about killing her mother are understood, not as part of normal Oedipal age sexual development, but rather as a legacy of Electra's extremely abusive

---

This work was partially funded by the Freida Brunn Fund, Milwaukee County Mental Health Complex. It is based on a paper presented at the Annual Meeting of the American Academy of Psychoanalysis in New York in May 1990 as the prize paper for the Esther Haar Award.

childhood. Electra's homicidal obsessions and compulsions express her intense rage toward her abusers. Anger, fears of anger dyscontrol, and episodes of inappropriate aggression or violence are part of the symptom pattern seen in victims of child abuse (Conte and Schuerman 1987; Donaldson and Gardner 1985; Goodwin 1987, 1989). Revenge fantasies are seen in other trauma victims, such as the "Rambo" fantasies in Vietnam veterans (Figley 1985) and fantasies of punishing the abuser in rape victims or in battered spouses (Ewing 1987; Gordon and Riger 1989; Katz and Mazur 1979; Ledray 1986). Also, children who have witnessed the murder of a parent fantasize about retaliating against the murderer (Pynoos and Eth 1985). Adult victims of multimodal child abuse complain of continuing intense anger at the perpetrator (Donaldson and Gardner 1985). Anger may be expressed in plans to escape the situation or bring the abuser to justice. Victims may displace their anger onto their current sexual partners or display antisocial behaviors in the form of child neglect, physical abuse of their children, arrests, and violence related to substance abuse (Goodwin et al. 1988; Russell 1986).

In this review, we retell the Electra myth as a story about obsessive revenge fantasies in a child abuse victim burdened by other posttraumatic symptoms as well. Electra's multimodal abuse history, her symptoms (e.g., anger dyscontrol, easy startle, unresolved grief, somatic symptoms), and qualities of her revenge fantasies and associated conspiracy to enact them will be compared to patterns from a recent case involving child abuse, parent loss, posttraumatic symptoms, revenge fantasies, and, ultimately, murder of the abusive parent.

The Case of Electra

Family and Abuse History

In mythology, and later in tragedies by Aeschylus (1959), Sophocles (1953), and Euripides (1959), Electra is described as the daughter of Agamemnon and Clytemnestra. Electra's own childhood abuse is listed as one episode in a long history of murder and even cannibalism of children practiced in her family, the House of Tantalus. More proximately, Agamemnon had killed Clytemnestra's first husband and all their children before taking her as his wife. Later, Agamemnon sacrificially killed his daughter, Iphigenia, to ensure success in his war against

Troy. Following his victory there, Agamemnon returned home with lovely Cassandra as his "trophy of war." Driven by hatred because of Agamemnon's murder of Iphigenia as well as his infidelity with Cassandra, Clytemnestra took Aegisthus as her lover, and together they conspired to murder Agamemnon. (Aegisthus also had an abusive background and was the product of father-daughter incest.) They also killed Cassandra and her twin sons by Agamemnon. Aegisthus then attempted to kill Orestes, Agamemnon's son, so that he would not inherit his father's throne. However, Orestes was rescued and taken into exile by one of Agamemnon's servants (whose own son was killed in Orestes' place).

After Agamemnon's death, the abuse of Electra becomes more pronounced. She is called a "worthless slut" by her mother, who prays that "the infernal gods will never deliver you from misery" (Sophocles 1953, p. 77). She is insulted ("you impudent creature") and threatened with abandonment ("you'll never see light, forever more, banished to end your life singing sad dirges in a vaulted dungeon") (p. 80). Electra becomes a virtual captive in her mother's palace: "Mother!—more like a jailer, with the slavery you put on me, the insults I have to bear from you and your partner . . . " (p. 86). She is prohibited from marrying, lest her offspring threaten Aegisthus's throne.

Electra's Symptoms

Electra's symptoms are described in some detail in the tragedies and overlap patterns identified in recent studies of child abuse victims.

Cinderella syndrome. The Cinderella syndrome has been described in abused children who later simulate or exaggerate neglect in a context of ongoing emotional abuse (Goodwin et al. 1980). Associated characteristics also found in Electra include the following:

1. Previous severe physical and/or sexual abuse or witnessed violence;
2. Unresolved grief over the early loss of a parental figure;
3. Feelings of helplessness and hopelessness; and
4. A mother figure who also has a history of abuse that interferes with her ability to help the child.

Children with this syndrome accuse their mothers of dressing them in rags, making them do all the chores, and favoring their step-siblings. Electra vividly describes her neglect and excess domestic duties in a lament truly reminiscent of the Cinderella tale: " . . . kept like a beast in stable rags, my skin heavy with grease and dirt. I weave my clothes myself and slavelike at the loom must work or else walk naked through the world in nothing. I am deprived of . . . dances" (Euripides 1959, p. 236). Her sister Chrysothemis chides Electra for making things worse than need be: "Have you not learnt after all this time to restrain your useless anger, not make a vain parade of it?" (Sophocles 1953, p. 78).

Like the children who experience the Cinderella syndrome, Electra was verbally and emotionally abused and experienced a strong sense of emotional abandonment: "Day in, day out, an endless summer of sorrow—hating and hated by my mother . . . " (Sophocles 1953, p. 76). Electra's earlier experiences of witnessed violence color the meaning of these insults; for her, the threat of death underlies them.

Electra's dramatic, unresolved grief over the death of her father, Agamemnon, is the central theme of her life and is eloquently expressed in the play. "How should misery not be endless? How could it every be better to forget the dead? Nature forbids it. That is no law for me" (Aeschylus 1959, pp. 75–76).

Her father's murderers are the only available parent figures. This exacerbates Electra's helplessness and hopelessness. At one point, Clytemnestra tries to explain her own victimization to Electra and how this prevents Clytemnestra from helping Electra mourn Agamemnon. However, Electra is not a receptive audience.

Depressive and somatic symptoms. Electra's hopelessness about her captive existence escalates to depression: "Half my life is wasted away in hopeless waiting; all my strength is gone" (Sophocles 1953, p. 74). Hopelessness is joined by other depressive symptoms: "My way is the way of the tearful bird . . . abandoned to despair . . . weeping eternally, with tears unceasing" (p. 73). Later, her despair escalates to suicidality when she comes to believe, falsely, that her brother has been killed: "Life is all pain to me, I want to die. If Orestes in his struggle falls to death, I too am dead, let them no longer say I live for I will stab my belly with a two-edged sword" (p. 93).

Close reading reveals Electra's somatic symptoms secondary to her self-neglect and depression. At one point Orestes comments to her,

"Sadness has wasted you so deeply I could weep." Electra replies, "I think you see me. First, my body wasted and dry. Next, my head razor-cropped like a victim of the Scythians" (Euripides 1959, p. 251). Whether her emaciation results only from depression or whether a separate eating disorder has supervened is not clear. Headache and easy startle are other symptoms. Electra's body tells the story of her misfortunes as eloquently as her words, emotions, and actions.

Qualities of Electra's Revenge Fantasies and Conspiracy

One appealing aspect of the revenge fantasy is that it allows Electra to treat her father's death as if it were reversible and as if he were still alive and able to accept her gift of revenge. She speaks to her sister as if their father were still living: "This is what you must give him: a lock of your own bright hair . . . and this of mine. In my poor state it is all I have to give. Kneel to him and pray that he himself will come from the dead to befriend us and help us against our enemies" (Sophocles 1953, p. 82).

Her fantasies of murdering Clytemnestra and Aegisthus are also a way for Electra to cope with her intolerable situation. Feeling frozen and helpless to act in reality, fantasy is her only outlet. In her depression, Electra's revenge fantasies allow her to redirect her anger outward at her abusers in order to relieve her own anger and guilt in a safer way than through suicide.

Knowing the family violence history, one might guess that originally Electra's anger was aimed both at Clytemnestra and Agamemnon. But, because of her need to have a good parent, Electra splits her anger and expresses it only toward the surviving Clytemnestra, while idealizing the dead (and now no longer threatening) Agamemnon. Electra's love, too, must once have belonged to both parents. It is her unconscious identification with Clytemnestra's homicidal solutions that fuels Electra's own homicidal fantasies and yet walls them off, outside of her awareness. Following Clytemnestra's death, Electra proclaims, "Behold, I wrap close in the robe, the one I loved, and could not love" (Euripides 1959, p. 393).

Because she is so paralyzed in her depression ("I can do nothing but wait in misery"; Sophocles 1953, p. 77), it is unlikely that Electra would have moved from fantasy to action on her own. However, the unexpected appearance of her brother Orestes allows her to move in small steps, first from fantasy to dialogue.

On the surface, Electra's conspiracy with Orestes to murder Clytemnestra seems calculated and well planned. But there is also a drivenness to Electra's dialogue and an inability to delay the moment of revenge or to consider the long-term consequences of her actions. Electra's derealization is so powerful that it is not clear if she realizes that she is entering an arena of action where the rules of fantasy and daydream no longer apply and where real consequences will ensue.

There also seems to be a contagiousness to her rage that infects Orestes. His own rage and agenda for violence accelerate as he is exposed to Electra's misery and pent-up fantasies. These revenge fantasies become one of the only vehicles for relatedness between this brother and sister who have had so little positive family relatedness that they are unable even to recognize one another upon first meeting.

What this family has taught both to do is share sadomasochistic fantasies, fantasies that involve homicide at one pole or double suicide at another. In versions of the play where Electra ends by marrying one of Orestes' companions, the sadomasochistic dialogue becomes as well the only vehicle of her erotic or romantic relatedness—the only way of life and love Electra has been taught.

When talking finally escalates to action, Electra is overcome by guilt in one version: "Weep greatly for me . . . for I am guilty. A girl flaming in hurt, I marched against the mother who bore me" (Euripides 1959, p. 256). In another version, there is even a feeling of surprise at the murder (Aeschylus 1959). It is as if the fantasies belong to Electra, but the deed itself is more central to the story of Orestes, who must now bear the moral and legal responsibility, while Electra is finally able to resolve her catastrophic reaction to the family trauma and go on with her life.

The Case of C.

Abuse and Family History

The following case history is drawn from public records (Kleiman 1988). C., a 15-year-old honor student and cheerleader, was physically, emotionally, and sexually abused by her father. When her younger sister reached the age at which C.'s sexual abuse began, C. started asking her brother and school friends how she might hire an assassin to kill her father. Her mother had died a year before, after many years of spousal abuse—a possible factor in the mother's final illness. All three siblings had been physically abused by their father with kicking and punching, often done in public. C. had received facial beatings, resulting in severe bruises and the inability to speak or eat for several days. One such beating occurred when her father found a valentine that C. had received. The father's use of an arsenal of guns, including automatic weapons, underlined his ability to carry out death threats. Discipline included yelling, screaming, and name-calling. The children were called "sissy" if they cried after the beatings, and C. was often called "whore" and "cunt."

C.'s sexual abuse began at age 11, progressing to intercourse at age 12. C.'s father told her that if she reported the sexual abuse, he would "beat her to death."

Both C.'s father and mother had also been physically and verbally abused in childhood and had witnessed violence.

C.'s Symptoms

Cinderella syndrome. After her mother died, C. became increasingly agitated about her abuse situation and became convinced that her younger sister was being sexually victimized. She felt a duty to her dead mother to protect this sister. As it turned out, C.'s fears about the sister were exaggerated. What was escalating in the somewhat protective mother's absence was C.'s own abuse—emotional, physical, and sexual.

C.'s premature assumption of responsibilities as wife and mother left her exhausted, especially since she was simultaneously trying to maintain a compensatory facade as a "perfect teenager." Her father's intrusiveness—prohibiting dating, going through her garbage and dresser drawers, and listening in on her telephone conversations—left C. as hindered as Cinderella in pursuing a normal social life.

C. was also unable to resolve her grief over her mother's death. C. felt guilty about having displaced her mother whom she now idolized and "prayed to," yet at the same time she felt anger toward her mother for abandoning her. C. heard her mother's voice and had visions of her. C. felt hopeless about halting the abuse in part because her mother, also a child abuse victim, had never been able to control her husband's abuse either of herself or of the children.

Depressive and somatic symptoms. C. felt powerless to stop her father's abuse for many reasons: his threats of retaliation; her commitment to her dead mother to maintain the family; and her resulting depression, manifested by weight loss, sleep disturbance, increasing fatigue, and suicidal thoughts. C. rejected suicide as a way out only because she felt that would leave her younger sister unprotected. When C. became pregnant (as it turned out, by a boyfriend, not by her father), her depressive and somatic symptoms increased as well as her panic.

Qualities of C.'s Revenge Fantasies

C.'s unresolved grief for her mother's death as well as her helplessness, guilt, fear, and anger about the incest prevented her from taking realistic action, a condition described by Summit (1983) as the "incest accommodation syndrome." Instead, C. began to formulate revenge fantasies in order to express her anger in a "safe" way. One may postulate that this anger was actually directed at both parents. But, in her need for an "ideal" parent, C. split her anger and expressed it only toward her surviving father, allowing a kind of loving imaginary companionship with her dead mother. For C., revenge was the only way she was able to justify to her mother her own unwilling participation in the sexual abuse.

As C.'s anger and fear intensified, so did her need to act on her revenge fantasies. However, her depressive immobilization led C. to recruit first her brother and then several classmates as the active agents of her fantasies. The revenge "plotting" served as an outlet for feelings of hurt, loss, and abandonment. C. found she could finally share these feelings with one of the adolescent classmates she approached. He also came from a violent family. Whenever their hurt threatened to surface, the "revenge talk" became more driven and insistent, the two coconspirators fostering each other's rage. When her classmate began to take action, C. reacted with a confusing mixture of delight, horror, surprise, and relief, alternately disavowing and embracing his action. In her derealization and mingling of fantasy with reality, C. was unable accurately to calculate the possible consequences of her revenge plans.

For C., the ultimate carrying out of the homicidal fantasy signalled entry into treatment and eventually a more normal life. No longer dominated by bitterness over her victimization, C. was able to pursue her subsequent marriage (to one of her more peripheral "coconspirators") and enter a professional career.

For the active coconspirator, the deed left him, like Orestes, at the mercy of the Furies, beset by both past and present problems and facing stiff legal penalties.

Discussion

Both Electra and C. experienced homicidal revenge fantasies and acted on them. As many as 70% of incest victims who seek treatment have experienced intrusive, repetitive fantasies of wanting to harm, castrate, or kill their perpetrator (Donaldson and Gardner 1985). One study of adult survivors of childhood incest and physical abuse who also experienced severe psychiatric symptoms showed that 4 of 10 had detailed plans to murder their perpetrator (Goodwin et al. 1988). However, it is rare that a victim of multimodal child abuse actually takes such action. Of the 89,000 murders committed in the United States from 1980–1984, only 2,266 were cases of completed parricide by victims of child abuse (Ewing 1990; Monas 1991).

More subtle forms of revenge fantasies are seen in other survivors of multimodal incestuous abuse. One woman said that she could not have done anything worse than what was already happening to her father: testicular cancer (Bass and Davis 1988). Such feelings can lead to catastrophic guilt when the perpetrator becomes ill or dies. Anger against men is another manifestation; one incest treatment group went to a male striptease show in order to "sadistically scrutinize the sexual endowment of the performers" and shout abusive comments (Ganzarin and Buchele 1987, p. 186).

The revenge sought by C. and Electra fits patterns of vengeance discussed by Socarides (1966). Unconsciously, the vengeful person attempts to conceal a damaged ego that resulted from being hurt and traumatized in childhood. Vengeance is a way to undo and deny the damage, to express the anger, and to persuade oneself that one need never fear deprivation or humiliation again.

Both C. and Electra expressed suicidal thoughts before committing the homicide. In a study by Monas (1991), 75% of child abuse victims who committed parricide expressed suicidal ideation within the 2 years prior to the homicide, and 50% expressed suicidal thoughts within 1 year afterward. Suicide as revenge against the perceived persecutor is aimed at disappointing, emotionally hurting, or inducing guilt. In effect it is "homicide turned against the self" and operates along the principles described by Socarides (1966; p. 373; Baechler 1975; Counts 1987; Hankoff and Einsidler 1979; Menninger 1959; Victoroff 1983).

These cases suggest that vengeful homicide or suicide is a risk when the following conditions exist:

1. Family violence is multiple and severe, involving multiple victims;
2. The victim has been through the loss of a trusted or idealized parent figure;
3. Posttraumatic symptoms are severe, especially those involving depression and feelings of helplessness; and
4. Dissociative symptoms and escape into fantasy are prominent defenses.

In addition the presence of an accomplice (even if imaginary or unwitting) (Morris 1982) seems a necessary, sometimes accidental, additional factor, one that may be essential in determining whether revenge obsessions remain in fantasy or enter the arena of action.

References

Aeschylus: Agamemnon and The Libation Bearers, in The Complete Greek Tragedies, Vol 1. Translated and edited by Grene D, Lattimore R. Chicago, IL, University of Chicago Press, 1959

Baechler J: Suicides. New York, Basic Books, 1975

Bass E, Davis L: The Courage to Heal. New York, Harper & Row, 1988

Conte J, Schuerman JR: Factors associated with an increased impact of child sexual abuse. Child Abuse Negl 11:201–211, 1987

Counts DA: Female suicide and wife abuse: a cross-cultural perspective. Suicide Life Threat Behav 17:194–204, 1987

Donaldson JA, Gardner R: Diagnosis and treatment of traumatic stress among women after childhood incest, in Trauma and Its Wake: The Study and Treatment of PTSD. Edited by Figley CR. New York, Brunner/Mazel, 1985, pp 356–377

Euripides: Electra, in The Complete Greek Tragedies, Vol 4. Translated and edited by Grene D, Lattimore R. Chicago, IL, University of Chicago Press, 1959

Ewing CP: Battered Women Who Kill: Psychological Self-Defense as a Legal Justification. Boston, MA, Lexington Books, 1987

Ewing CP: When Children Kill: The Dynamics of Juvenile Homicide. Boston, MA, Lexington Books, 1990

Figley CR (ed): Trauma and Its Wake: The Study and Treatment of Post-Traumatic Stress Disorder. New York, Brunner/Mazel, 1985

Freud S: The psychogenesis of a case homosexuality in a woman (1920), in The Standard Edition of the Complete Psychological Works of Sigmund Freud, Vol 18. Translated and edited by Strachey J. London, Hogarth Press, pp 146–174, 1955

Ganzarin R, Buchele B: Acting out during group psychotherapy for incest. Int J Group Psychother 37:185–200, 1987

Goodwin J: Development impacts of incest, in Handbook of Child Psychiatry, Vol V. Edited by Noshpitz D, Berlin J, Call I, et al. New York, Basic Books, 1987, pp 103–110

Goodwin J: Sexual Abuse: Incest Victims and Their Families. Chicago, IL, Year Book Medical, 1989

Goodwin J, Cauthorne CG, Rada RT: Cinderella syndrome: children who simulate neglect. Am J Psychiatry 137:1223–1225, 1980

Goodwin J, Cheeves K, Connell V: Defining a syndrome of severe symptoms in survivors of severe incestuous abuse. Dissociation 1:11–16, 1988

Gordon MT, Riger S: The Female Fear. New York, Free Press, 1989

Hankoff LD, Einsidler B: Suicide: Theory and Clinical Aspects. Ann Arbor, MI, Books on Demand, 1979

Jung C: The theory of psychoanalysis, in The Collected Works of C. G. Jung, Vol 4. New York, Bollingen Foundation, 1961, pp 83–228

Katz S, Mazur M: Understanding the Rape Victim: A Synthesis of Research Findings. New York, Wiley, 1979

Kleiman D: A Deadly Silence: A Case of Incest and Murder. New York, Atlantic Monthly Press, 1988

Ledray LE: Recovering From Rape. New York, Henry Holt, 1986

Menninger K: A Psychiatrist's World. New York, Viking, 1959

Monas P: When a Child Kills: Abused Children Who Kill Their Parents. New York, Simon & Schuster, 1991

Morris M: If I Should Die Before I Wake. Los Angeles, CA, JP Tarcher, 1982

Pynoos RS, Eth S: Developmental perspective on psychic trauma in childhood, in Trauma and Its Wake: The Study and Treatment of Post-Traumatic Stress Disorder, Edited by Figley CR. New York, Brunner/Mazel, 1985, pp 36–52

Russell D: The Secret Trauma: Incest in the Lives of Girls and Women. New York, Basic Books, 1986

Socarides CW: On vengeance: the desire to get even. J Am Psychoanal 14:356–375, 1966

Sophocles: Electra and Other Plays. Translated by Watling EF. London, Penguin, 1953

Summit R: The child sexual abuse accommodation syndrome. Child Abuse Negl 7:177–193, 1983

Victoroff V: The Suicidal Patient: Recognition, Intervention, Management. Montvale, NJ, Medical Economics Books, 1983

Section II

Exorcism and Possession States

Replacing yesterday's misconceptions with today's is not always an advance.

Stuart Schneiderman, *Rat Man*

I am toying with the idea that in the perversions . . . we may have the remnants of a primitive sexual cult, which . . . may once have been a religion.

Sigmund Freud, *The Complete Letters of Sigmund Freud to Wilhelm Fliess (1877–1904)*

The unconscious is always cultural and when it talks it tells you your old stories, it tells you the old stories you've heard before because it consists of the repressed of culture. But it is also always shaped by the forceful return of a libido that doesn't give up that easily, and also by what is strange, what is outside culture, by a language which is a savage tongue, that can make itself understood quite well.

Helene Cixous, "Castration or Decapitation?", *Signs,* 7

Editor's Introduction

Together with Freud and Janet, whose cases are discussed in this section, the authors of this book view "possession" as the cultural category into which severe posttraumatic syndromes have been placed throughout most of human history and in many different cultures. Because this conceptualization was so widespread in the Middle Ages and at the time of Freud's seventeenth-century "case," and because medieval concepts dominate the patients' imagery even in the present-day cases, I have placed this material on possession here, between the Greeks and the French Revolution, despite the fact that Freud and Janet themselves belong, quite thoroughly, to the nineteenth century.

Both chapters on possession deal with ancient questions that remain unanswered. What is the disturbance of the self that human beings convey through the symbolism of possession? How is it that exorcism rituals sometimes seem to repair this intrusion or distortion in the self?

These two chapters approach these questions in different ways. The first one, following Freud, emphasizes decoding the symbolic meanings of the possessing entity and the symptoms produced by the demon in order to reconstruct a narrative of the patient's life experience. Ultimately one uncovers the unconscious wishes and fears that made that original narrative unacceptable to memory and so allowed the demonic narrative to become its substitute. In the case of the seventeenth-century exorcism, Freud reconstructed the death of a father and subsequent pathological mourning with regression to feminine identifications. We rework this decoding, reconstructing sadistic abuse as well as abandonment, and illustrate how similar life circumstances led a present-day patient to seek out exorcism, again with surprisingly helpful results.

In the second chapter, based on Janet's case, the emphasis is on the unique qualities of the mental state entered by such traumatized individuals. All the qualities of hypnotizability are described: the dream-like quality of cognition, the use of body and action language, the suggestibility, the ability to experience a doubling of consciousness, the ability to experience and observe simultaneously or experience in multiple modes simultaneously, the capacity for active imagery, and the creation of fantasy worlds. Witztum and van der Hart describe an elegant brief treatment of such a case illustrating how much progress can be made by working with the positive creative aspects of this state rather than trying to medicate or intimidate the patient out of trance and into a state the therapist may prefer or experience as "normal."

Still another way to analyze possession and exorcism is to examine the techniques of exorcism. In an earlier publication, Sally Hill and I described seven techniques common to most exorcism traditions: 1) careful attention to diagnosis, 2) use of ritual objects and sacred space, 3) use of incantations and music, 4) attention to body position and holding, 5) confrontation, 6) attention to risks to the exorcist, and 7) attention to aftercare and relapse prevention (Hill and Goodwin 1989). We asked whether these commonalities in evolved techniques might relate to core characteristics of that subgroup of traumatized individuals whose symptoms are so severe as to compel treatment intervention.

The trauma-based symptom that seemed to account for the attentiveness to diagnosis so characteristic of traditional exorcisms was the tendency in victims toward concealment, both of prior victimization and of current symptoms, because of the coerced secrecy that surrounds human-inflicted trauma. The focus on physical rather than human objects we connected with the deep mistrust victimized children acquire for human beings. We saw the use of chants and music as effective ways to communicate with individuals experiencing traumatic trance states. The emphasis on the body makes sense if one assumes that traumatic memories often are encoded more as body sensations than as verbal mental content. The emphasis on confrontation is necessary when trying to free a patient from the grip of a repetition compulsion reinforced in the child by multiple adult abusers and in the adult by repeated reenactments of violent conflicts. The confronting therapist is at risk, because the victim carries within her in some form the introjected victimizer and will reenact all aspects of her struggle in victimizer as well as victim roles. Relapse is a risk; new life events may trigger aspects of the trauma complex that have not yet been verbally recalled and worked through, and symptoms may have blocked or distorted much of normal development, which must now be resumed and relearned.

The imagery of possession remains central for victims of sadistic abuse. The abuser has treated the child as his or her possession, important only insofar as the abuser can exploit the child to satisfy his or her desires. For many victims, it is an alien concept that one might live other than as a slave—as if one's life were one's own possession, as if one's own viewpoint and desires had intrinsic merit. Such victims continue to hear and obey the abuser's voice either literally or figuratively.

The "demons" treat the patient in the same way the abuser did, reviling, vandalizing, mutilating (often genitally). Other symptom complexes, more familiar to our late twentieth-century cultural paradigms, allow similar reenactments of sadistic tyranny. Alcohol/substance abuse, severe eating disorders, and borderline syndromes are engines of pain in themselves and can lead also to treatment in which the victim is once again locked up, tied down, forcibly drugged or fed, and emotionally abused. Such treatments, like exorcism, can become no more than another reenactment of the sadistic abuse unless continual efforts are made to interpret and transform the repetitions.

Perversion, discussed in the next section, may be seen as the triumph of the possessing sadistic abuser—the killing of all pleasure in the victim, substituting for spontaneity, pleasure, and love the endless enactments of the abuses, with the victimized person now fully entered and replaced by his or her abuser. This is the stage of "I love Big Brother" described in *1984* by Orwell, whose own life experience of victimization had taught him much (Shengold 1989).

Theoretical and clinical questions remain. What causes the loss of ego boundaries that characterizes "Stockholm syndrome" and the more drastic incorporations described here of fragments of the abuser's likes, dislikes, ideals, motives, and behaviors? A psychodynamic answer would focus on the child's wish for an intact parent, which is more intense than the wish for a self. The child allows the parent into him- or herself in order to be protected and improved. Then there are the death fears, which can be escaped by abandoning the victimized self and becoming (in fantasy) someone else. Janet would remind us, too, that one core characteristic of trance is uncritical hypersuggestibility, so that the derogatory emotional abuse by the abuser and his or her demands for total control enter the victim's awareness entirely unscreened and ready to be acted on.

Both modern cases described in this section map therapeutic paths back to a more boundaried experience of self, freed from enslavement and possession by the abuser.

References

Hill S, Goodwin JM: Satanism: similarities between patient accounts and pre-Inquisition historical sources. Dissociation 2:39–44, 1989

Shengold L: Soul Murder: The Effects of Childhood Abuse and Deprivation. New Haven, CT, Yale University Press, 1989

Chapter 3

Freud's Notes on a Seventeenth-Century Case of Demonic Possession: Understanding the Uses of Exorcism

Sally Hill, M.S.W.
Jean M. Goodwin, M.D., M.P.H.

Exorcism is an ancient form of treatment for mental illness usually connected to folk beliefs that psychopathology is caused by spirits of the dead, possession by demons, or influence by other foreign bodies or intelligences. Diagnostic criteria for possession are remarkably similar cross-culturally and resemble symptoms described in Western medical culture as dissociative (Davis 1980; Goodman 1988). "Possession state" has been suggested as an addition to the dissociative disorder section of the next Diagnostic Statistical Manual (Saxena and Prasad 1989). In the United States, dissociative patients who also have been involved with satanic cults may seek exorcism from clergy concurrently with psychotherapy, thereby propelling the therapist to become educated about exorcism as it is practiced in the Judeo-Christian tradition (Hill and Goodwin 1989). Some theorists both from psychology and anthropology have suggested that the historically ancient and cross-culturally ubiquitous techniques for exorcism may have applications for those clinicians treating dissociative patients within contemporary paradigms (Allison 1980; Goodman 1988).

In this chapter, we compare Freud's understanding of a seventeenth-century case of demon possession and exorcism with a modern case of a patient who had been involved in a satanic cult and had experienced demon possession, and who sought out exorcism as well as psychotherapy.

Freud's Analysis of a Seventeenth-Century Case

According to Strachey, Freud had a long-standing interest in witchcraft and possession. He translated an 1886 lecture by Charcot on a sixteenth-century case of possession and discussed these topics in two letters to Fliess (1897/1954, Letters 56 and 57). In 1923, Freud published his analysis of a seventeenth-century painter whose possession and two exorcisms had been described in brief letters from the referring and exorcising priests and in the painter's own illustrated diary.

On August 29, 1677, a Bavarian native, Johann Christoph Haizmann, suddenly began to experience convulsions in the chapel of the castle of Pottenbrunn in Lower Austria, where he was employed as a painter. These convulsions persisted, and he was questioned by the chapel prefect, who asked if Haizmann had been practicing forbidden arts or had entered into a pact with the devil. The painter, after asking everyone else to leave the room, confessed to the prefect that he had indeed sold himself to the devil 9 years previously, after the death of a relative, and now feared that the devil was coming for him. He insisted that the devil could only be forced to return their signed pact at Mariazell, the Shrine of the Most Blessed Virgin Mary, in nearby Styria. He resolved to go there, arriving September 5. After 3 days and nights of continued exorcism by priests from the Convent of St. Lambert, at midnight on the Feast of the Nativity, Haizmann retrieved the pact from the devil, who had appeared to him at the altar.

Apparently cured, the painter was sent to Vienna to live with a married sister. There he joined the Rosicrucians; a month later, however, beginning October 11, between 11 and 12 at night, he was again plagued by convulsions, trance states, and visions of various demons. He experienced these demons interfering with his sleep and with his prayers and confession, torturing him with ropes, excessive heat and stench, and feverish shivering. In his visions, the painter saw well-dressed cavaliers, often with beautiful women, inviting him to partake in earthly pleasures, to come and be their king, and urging him to destroy his paintings. He saw "harlots' pranks and lewd practices" in these visions and described "everything" as "topsy-turvy." In addition, the painter reported visions of heavenly personalities who both appealed to him with scenes of eternal bliss and threatened him with eternal damnation, as they tried to persuade him to become a hermit.

This continued for almost 7 months until May 1678, at which time

Haizmann returned to the Shrine of the Virgin Mary. He then told of a second pact he had made with the devil, this one signed with his own blood. Again, exorcism was performed until the devil returned the second pact, on May 9.

Haizmann then settled into a religious life of relative peace, joining the Brothers Hospitallers and taking the name Chrysostomus. He died 22 years later, on March 14, 1700, of a "slow fever" in Neustatt in Bohemia.

Freud's Interpretation

Freud saw possession states as neuroses and demons as unacceptable wishes repressed and projected onto the external world. In Freud's analysis, Christoph Haizmann was experiencing a melancholic depression precipitated by his father's death and complicated by work inhibition and anxiety about the future (1923/1953). The devil became a father substitute toward whom the painter had conflicting feelings. The bond with the devil was a "neurotic fantasy" through which the painter expressed his ambivalence. The painter longed for his father, both because of material need and because an earlier strong fixation on his mother had been displaced onto the father. This longing awakened in the painter a repressed feminine position toward his father—a homosexual wish, including the fantasy of becoming pregnant by him. However, this implied castration and was therefore unacceptable, making the father a terrifying figure. In making the pact with the devil, the painter hoped to regain what he had lost by obtaining a father substitute, while also debasing the feared father by portraying him as demonic and (in some of his paintings) as feminine.

This solution was not successful for Haizmann, because he succumbed again to melancholia and became unable to work. He thus turned for assistance to the Holy Mother as well as to several fathers (priests). When the first exorcism was unsuccessful, Freud hypothesizes that the painter fabricated the second bond (1923/1953). The second exorcism was not the curative factor, however; instead, joining a Holy Order ended both Haizmann's financial and internal struggles.

Freud (1923/1953) concludes that perhaps Haizmann was unable to pull himself away from his mother's breast; throughout life, he demanded to be nourished by someone else, a demand that he met by becoming a monk and being cared for by fathers, albeit sacrificing most of the possibilities of enjoyment in life. The demon possession, to Freud, resulted from the failure of the painter to successfully resolve the Oedipal conflict, remaining in the feminine, homosexual position toward his father. The devil was both a father substitute and a condensed symbol of Haizmann's conflictual libidinal wishes toward his father.

Macalpine and Hunter's Interpretation

Reviewing the case a half-century after Freud, Macalpine and Hunter (1956) came to different conclusions. They translate the term "ex morte parentis" in the original text to mean only that someone in the painter's family died; the phrase does not specify the precise relationship to the painter of the dead relative. The authors wonder if Freud assumed it was the father because Freud's own interest in demonology began a few months after his own father's death. They go on to question Freud's conclusion that Haizmann experienced conflicting, homosexual feelings toward his father, pointing out that there is no direct mention either of homosexuality or of the father in the painter's diary.

In addition, Macalpine and Hunter (1956) challenge Freud's explanation for the feminine characteristics in Haizmann's devils as evidence of mother-fixation. Freud (1923/1953) stated that it was unusual to find the devil portrayed with feminine characteristics. However, the later authors were able to cite many such depictions of devils. In fact, the presence of supernumerary breasts, as seen in Haizmann's devil, was a well-known characteristic of witches.

Macalpine and Hunter (1956) see the problems of the painter as primarily pregenital and thus inextricably attached to erroneous ideas about sexuality and reproduction. They point out that the idea of the devil as it has evolved contains many bisexual features that resonate with pregenital positions. The devil originated from serpent and dragon images, symbols of creation and fertility, encompassing all of reproduction with both feminine and masculine principles. They point to the lack of genital differentiation in the paintings as evidence of the painter's pregenital fixation, in which he fantasizes being both male and female—being a boy, but a boy who might also have a baby. Macalpine and Hunter hypothesize that the precipitant may have been not the death of Haizmann's father but his sister's having a baby, thereby depriving the painter of sole access to her maternal care and challenging his procreation fantasies.

In this view, the painter experienced confusion about sexual identity and procreation, with no appreciation for the role of sex in reproduction. His convulsions were hypochondriacal delusions and hallucinations, connected to fantasies of giving birth, being born, dying, and being reborn. These "body fantasies" were not able to be verbalized. The pacts with the devil are seen as a "rationalization by which the painter attempted to account for the terrible expectations of impending life and death which he experienced" (Macalpine and Hunter 1956, p. 112).

Haizmann's improvement after the first exorcism Macalpine and Hunter (1956) attribute to submission to the Holy Virgin (i.e., recognition of the biological reality that only women can bear children). This enabled him to identify with men, shown in his religious vocation, having "surrendered his female identification to the Holy Mother" (p. 113). However, the male identification required the renunciation of sexual reproduction. Macalpine and Hunter believed that the painter's illness was too severe to be accounted for in terms of a homosexual conflict. Instead, they traced the illness to a pregenital quest for bisexuality symbolized by the pact with the devil, which is finally relinquished.

A Posttraumatic Interpretation

Another possibility, based on contemporary experience with patients who consider themselves possessed by demons, would be that Christoph Haizmann had experienced severe sadistic abuse. Such survivors often cannot give a direct account of their extreme abuse because terror and amnesia block internal narration and verbalization.

Seventeenth-century Bavaria offered a variety of violent and malevolent contexts that may have affected this case. Most obviously, given his possession diagnosis, Haizmann would have been concerned about involvement with the Inquisition, which had executed 274 witches in Bavaria in 1629 (including children under 5) and which continued to use torture as an interrogation technique until 1806 (Trevor-Roper 1968). Haizmann's involvement with the Rosicrucians, a Christian esoteric sect centered on alchemy, would have increased his anxieties in this regard. Lower Austria's inquisitorial mania came later than Bavaria's and was at its peak in the 1670s, when Haizmann's symptoms came to the notice of the church (R.J.W. Evans 1979).

Another significant factor would have been the Thirty Years' War, which devastated Germany from 1618 to 1648. Bavaria was occupied from 1645 to 1648, and some villages lost as much as two-thirds of their population (Parker 1984; Steinberg 1967). We do not know how old Haizmann was when he fell ill in 1668, but we know he was established as an artist. If he was in his late twenties then, he would have had firsthand exposure in childhood to the horrors chronicled in the picaresque novel *Simplicissimus,* published in 1668 (Grimmelshausen 1670/1964, 1668/1989), and later used by Brecht as the basis for his play "Mother Courage" (Brecht 1970). An invasion by the French in 1668 triggered fears in some survivors of the war that the devastation would begin again.

Certainly Haizmann's parents would have been directly exposed to the Thirty Years' War. Plague and famine, so severe as to lead to cannibalism, were major sources of civilian mortality. Bavaria's Oberammergau passion play was initiated in these years in thanksgiving for that village's relative deliverance from the plague (Ergang 1956). Marauding bands of soldiers raped, killed, and pillaged, set fire to villages, and tortured civilians at random (Benecke 1978; Wedgwood 1938). Military justice involved mass public hangings of deserters. Even after the truce, these bands persisted as criminal gangs; one such bandit was convicted in 1654 for more than 250 murders, including cannibalistic ones (Ergang 1956). Prostitution followed the armies—with a gentrified difference in the seventeenth century, as courtesans became the fashionable companions for the mercenary cavaliers fighting in the religious wars (H. Evans 1979).

Family violence must have been present in seventeenth-century Bavaria; contemporary records from Essex, England, indicate that more than half of homicides in this era involved parents killing their children (Cockburn 1977). Family violence has been documented in a contemporary possession case, that of Elizabeth Knapp, who was exorcised in New England in 1671 (Demos 1982). Like Haizmann, Elizabeth presented with pseudoseizures, visions, and somatic symptoms. Like him, she confessed a pact with the devil and underwent multiple exorcisms. Recent research into her genealogy reveals multiple criminal complaints against her father for adultery and drunkenness and an apparent psychotic breakdown in her mother after the death of an infant.

In Haizmann's context, all of these sources of violence would have been interactive: the religious wars intensified the interest in and the propaganda value of the demon possessed (Walker 1981). Increased violence led to an increased demand for revenge magic, and more prostitution led to more practice of love magic; both were major targets of the Inquisition. Crime, family violence, and mental illness probably increased in tandem in the aftermath of war. As Grimmelshausen's character Courage notes, "In war most people become worse, rather than better" (1670/1964, p. 21).

Many of the painter's symptoms resemble those seen in survivors of sadistic abuse. The painter describes "absences" and "trances," after which he would "come back" to himself. These suggest dissociative episodes. In these states, he describes visions and voices and undergoes what may be pseudoseizures. Some hallucinations could be understood as flashback material (e.g., the cavaliers and sexually inviting ladies representing fragmented memories of group sexual experiences). Other content such as a cauldron full of human bodies, people dancing in a circle, and a book of black magic, as well as some of the dates of symptomatic worsening (Lammas Day, the October Satanic High Holidays, Christmas, May Day) suggest a pseudoreligious satanic pattern in the reexperienced sadistic material (see Chapter 5). Some of these images—the cauldron of human bodies, the courtesans and cavaliers, the encounters with dangerous vagabonds—could be specific to Haizmann's wartime experiences.

Pseudoseizures for many survivors involve somatic reexperiencing of sexual abuse memories (Goodwin, in press). They may occur together with true seizures, because neurological and psychological trauma coincide when a child is sadistically maltreated. Haizmann's description of bleeding from the nose and mouth as a result of the violent thrashing in his convulsions is suggestive of the self-mutilation sometimes found in the pseudoseizures of sadistic abuse survivors. Another typical feature of pseudoseizures is that they occur in a public, symbolic setting (such as in church) as well as when the patient is alone.

Other somatic symptoms suggest victimization. At times, Haizmann described a stench and intense heat; these could represent flashback sensations or autonomic reexperiencing of traumatic sexual episodes. Shivering is a symptom seen in many rape victims that is sometimes traceable to somatic memories of being left unclothed and outdoors after the sexual assault. Sleep disturbance is a common symptom in children who were awakened to be abused. The painter's description of the demons torturing him with ropes could represent a somatic memory of bondage, a flashback (perhaps to witnessed hangings or other tortures), or self-mutilation inflicted by a dissociated self-fragment.

There are some signs of ego disintegration in Haizmann. Some of the hallucinated personages such as the hermit, Christ on the cross, angels, and radiant light seem to function as visualized imaginary friends or protective self-fragments. The demons who sat on the painter's tongue, the voices telling him to destroy his pictures of what he experienced and to become a hermit—all could be seen as internalized representations of the abusers' threats still interfering with his revealing the secrets about his victimization. In at least one contemporary seventeenth-century case, criminals cut out the tongue of a child witness to a murder (Marshburn 1971).

Haizmann's paintings themselves depict progressive sexual escalations that parallel those described by pedophiles and their victims: the devil (abuser) appears initially as an ordinary man, fully clothed and friendly, but progressively becomes less human and less fully clothed. In the final depiction, the devil is portrayed with grotesquely prominent genitals.

In addition, the painter shows other symptoms commonly seen in abuse survivors. He has an affective disorder with melancholia and sleep disturbance, severe guilt and shame, and possible substance abuse (one description states he was more likely to have episodes when he had a bit too much wine; this observation of exacerbation would be found also in true seizures).

Age of onset in adulthood is typical. Dissociative amnesia tends to break down in this developmental phase; it is more difficult to cover symptoms as secondary to alcohol use or "wild oats." If this is a case involving childhood trauma, either the death of an abuser or the loss of a supportive figure could have triggered symptoms. Aspects of severe victimization missing in this case include evidence of an eating disorder; physical, documentary, or medical evidence of abuse (the pacts and drawings seem more analogous to present-day data from patient journals and drawings); and witness testimony. However, absence of an explicit violence history is characteristic of such cases as they were described up to about 1900 (See Chapter 6); Freud's Dora case (Chapter 8) is one of the first in which a violence history was elicited and connected to symptoms.

Working from this hypothesis, we would assume that the symptomatic improvement observed after the exorcisms resulted from specific effects on the painter's posttraumatic symptoms. These psychodynamics will be discussed in detail in reference to the contemporary case presented later in this chapter. Entry into the monastery likely stabilized the painter's situation because of 1) decreased sexual triggers for post–sexual abuse symptoms, 2) stabilization of basic functions such as eating and sleeping, and 3) adoption of a new name and identity, which may have allowed a less costly form of dissociative adaptation.

The name that Haizmann adopted, Chrysostomus, literally means "golden-tongued" and refers to a fifth-century saint, John Chrysostom, who was famed for his eloquent denunciations of licentious displays in the imperial games and of prostitutes, including the empress. Because of his insistence on speaking out, John Chrysostom was sent into exile as a hermit.

A Contemporary Case

We now examine a contemporary case, a patient who experienced demon possession and underwent exorcism rituals concurrently with psychotherapy. In this instance, the history of sadistic abuse was well-documented and available to the therapist.

Barbara, a 42-year-old college-educated advertising executive, entered treatment after her brother confronted family members about his sexual abuse at the hands of their grandfather, who had recently separated from the family. This led to Barbara's realizing she had been abused by this relative also.

Barbara and her husband reported that her behavior and personality had been erratic for many years. At times she spoke, acted, and thought as a child. At other times she experienced herself as a very "bad" delinquent teenager; on still other occasions, she felt like an adult woman. Her thought patterns, responses, and reactions varied greatly, depending on her state.

During the course of treatment, eight "parts" of Barbara emerged, each with his or her own age, characteristics, and memories of childhood. A diagnosis of Dissociative Disorder Not Otherwise Specified was made.

Hypnosis aided Barbara in the recollection of severe sadistic emotional, physical, and sexual abuse from before age 2 through adolescence. Abuse was connected with participation in meetings of a satanic cult group. Her grandfather was the primary perpetrator of the abuse, involving her in oral, anal, and vaginal intercourse; sexual abuse took place, often with one or more adult coperpetrators and with other child victims. Sadistic elements included the witnessed killing of animals and humans, being buried until unconscious, and being impregnated, with ritual aborting of the fetus. In addition to the patient and her brother, three other family members described involvement in these sadistic practices, which were not recognized or acknowledged in any way during "normal" family life.

During treatment, Barbara began to report that she was oppressed or possessed by demons. Hypnotic exploration revealed a demon given to her by her grandfather as a gift and a companion during childhood. Barbara drew a picture of this demon for the therapist and recalled how her grandfather told her the creature would know if she revealed the secrets of the sadistic abuse, and then would tell him about her betrayal. Throughout her childhood, the demon would appear unpredictably and tease Barbara, taunting her, laughing at her, and moving her possessions so that she could not find them. Barbara spoke of later demons sent by her grandfather and the satanic cult group to oppress her; these demons would call her names, attack her self-confidence, augment her suicidal and homicidal thoughts, and generally undermine and torment her.

Barbara was very involved in religion and sought help from clergy regarding her experiences. She elected to participate in several exorcisms in order to rid herself of the demons' influence; this included several follow-up consultations.

The therapist's original position was one of alarm, with an effort to explore the meanings within the treatment of this seemingly irrational request. However, because the patient was intent on this course, the therapist, when asked, agreed to witness two of the patient's exorcisms. To the therapist's surprise, the interactions involved a calm and gentle verbal calling out of the "demons," a questioning about their perceived right to exist in the patient, a revocation of the grounds for that perceived right, and finally a formal expelling of the "demons." The clergyman helped Barbara and her husband learn to use this process on their own, as in this theological scheme, laypersons as well as clergy have access to the power needed to expel demons.

Theoretical Understanding of the Patient's Demons

Barbara described her experience of the internal demons as follows:

> I often feel as though someone or something else is controlling my thoughts and feelings. There is an almost constant barrage of negative self feelings that I have to suppress in order to get anything done. "You're no good. You're a fat, ugly slob. You have no discipline. Everyone's laughing at you. You don't fit in anywhere." I mostly feel powerless to stop the barrage. I feel there is a hold on me that has been there perhaps since birth. This something doesn't want me to succeed in life. I want to soar; this thing is working hard to keep my wings clipped. It goes against what I otherwise know about myself. I don't feel like I fit in my current body or my current life, yet I'm unable to change either one—someone else is controlling both of those areas. As soon as I decide to change any one of these areas, the barrage begins. It washes over me until I run back in the corner and hide, begging it to stop. I've become afraid to make any moves for fear of the beating that follows.

On a symbolic level, we understood her demons as representing five different aspects of her abuse experience. The first two listed below are similar to Freud's understanding of Haizmann, only deepened by the detailed history we have of this patient's abuse.

Demons as internalized abusers. One way to see Barbara's demons is as internalized introjects of the aggressors. Identification with the aggressor is a familiar mechanism in the normal development of the superego (A. Freud 1966). It is the process through which a child internalizes criticism from others of his or her behavior, thereby developing the capacity for self-criticism. The possessing demons can be viewed as internalizations of the abusers' criticisms, resulting in an extremely harsh self-critical agency. In a healthy process of identification with the aggressor, the internalized criticism becomes a standard required by the superego and comes to match the ego's evaluation of a fault. Because Barbara had dissociated the abuse, she could not recognize the harsh criticism as the sadistic and degrading voice of her grandfather. Instead, she experienced the demons as correctly assessing her value. As a result, Barbara suffered (as do many sadistic abuse survivors) from a highly distorted sense of guilt, which was not consonant with her behaviors and was therefore beyond the ego's capacity to resolve.

Identification with the aggressor is also a mechanism for dealing with anxiety. "By impersonating the aggressor, assuming his attributes or imitating his aggression, the child transforms himself from the person threatened into the person who makes the threat" (A. Freud 1966, p. 113). In this sense, Barbara identified with her abusers by incorporating them as her demons, thereby warding off painful victimization experiences of helplessness and degradation.

Experiencing the demons as partially inside but also partially outside herself allowed Barbara to avoid the painful experiencing of her complete helplessness as a victim, but without requiring the kind of seamless introjection that might have led to her becoming a sadistic abuser herself.

Demons as libidinal gratifications. A second function of Barbara's demons is to embody the gratifications available in the sadomasochistic activities, including sexual stimulation, discharge outlets for murderous aggression and rage, and competitive success, as gaining preference from her grandfather. Some of Barbara's demons were given names such as Murder, Lust, and Greed. At that stage, the demons were identified with unacceptable wishes, but as more libidinal energies were reclaimed, modified versions of these experiences became acceptable gratifications.

Demons as keepers of the secret. As illustrated in Barbara's description, a third way to view the demons is as "created" alters suggested by sadistic perpetrators sophisticated enough to use traumatic dissociation for the purpose of monitoring or enforcing compliance and secrecy. It is as effective to give children posthypnotic suggestions in traumatically induced dissociative states as after other types of hypnotic inductions. Barbara once described the watchful "companion" her grandfather gave her as the "inside of Granddad."

Demons as protectors. The demons serve a fourth function—self-preservation and protection. They contain Barbara's own knowledge about how to comply with the explicit and implicit rules of the sadistic group, thereby helping her to minimize her exposure to their abuse.

Demons as substitutes for memory. Finally, the demons serve as a substitute for memory. The demons provide a pseudoexplanation for Barbara's emotional pain while helping her to avoid the painful recognition that it is really her grandfather's voice she is hearing. Because remembering the abuse would be overwhelming and dangerous, both internally and externally, the demons allow Barbara to have some capacity for aggression, some libidinal gratification, and enough self-protective knowledge to comply with the abusers, while keeping the secret and bypassing the need for narrative memory of the abuse.

Understanding the Utility of Exorcism in the Modern Case

In other patients we have seen, exorcism experiences have proved quite toxic; the patient felt blamed by the exorcist or felt vital parts of the self were being expelled or labeled as bad. However, in Barbara's case, as in the case of Christoph Haizmann, symptoms seemed to improve rather than worsen. Like Freud, we become interested in explaining this.

The use of clerical exorcism along with psychotherapy seemed to address the five internal functions for demons described in the previous section. First, the clerical exorcist insists that the demon reveal his master and motivations, and in this process clarifies that the demon does not belong in the self system of the patient. The exorcism process makes explicit that the demon represents the aggressor. For Barbara, it helped bring her self-concept into line with her current beliefs—that she is a child of God who is not responsible for what happened to her. The exorcist identifies the demon as part of the aggressor, attempting to remove the introjected self-blame by identifying it as a viewpoint belonging to the aggressor, not to the victim. This has been particularly helpful to Barbara, as her grandfather had an impeccable reputation as a fine, upstanding citizen; and so, in her perception, no one, not even Barbara herself, could believe that he was a sadistic rapist. It was easier to believe that the problem was inside her. The exorcism identifies the abusers as she experienced them, so cruel as to forfeit human status. As with the demons, this extreme level of interpersonal attack cannot be accommodated or rationalized but must be extruded or fled from.

Secondly, the exorcism allows the victim to reexperience the powerful emotions associated with the dissociated trauma in a new mode that is not sadomasochistic. Reexternalizing the sadism from internal demons to her abusers means that Barbara can identify the abusers as the sadists and herself as the victim, thus rejecting sadism as a part of her. In so doing, she can acknowledge her own helpless, rageful, and overstimulated responses to the experience, while distinguishing these responses from her abusers' violence, sadism, and sociopathy. For Barbara, this differentiation heralded the appearance of alters who are able to express anger; before, this emotion had been avoided completely, because Barbara was so afraid she would express it in sadistic attacks.

The exorcist's personal role also helped Barbara differentiate sadists from nonsadists. The exorcist was a man who helped protect her, who identified her abusers as evil, and who perceived them as not a part of her. He assumed the position of a "good enough" father representing God, an all-powerful father who has authority over all creatures. Her past experience had been that only those who hurt have power; she had had to be emotionally and physically hurt in order to be gratified, especially with a man. In the exorcism, Barbara experienced ritual, spiritual, authoritative, and trance elements of empowerment and contact, but she did not have to be hurt. Fairbairn (1943/1954b) described this aspect of treatment in a brief comment on Freud's analysis of the Haizmann case: "The analytic treatment of Christoph [Haizmann] would be a formidable task . . . the appeal of a good object is indispensable in promoting a dissolution of the cathexes of internalized bad objects" (p. 74).

The created demonic alters are identified in the exorcism process as being the creatures of the abusers, not the agents of Barbara. It becomes more clear that the created alters are intrusions created for the convenience of the abusers in order to produce compliance and secrecy.

In addition, the exorcism process makes explicit that the demons' advice regarding self-protection was appropriate within the sadistic group, but not in other contexts. The perpetrators had described the demon alter as a companion, someone to help Barbara follow the rules; the exorcist helped her recognize that the demon's help was not based on the patient's best interests but on the needs of the sadistic group. As Barbara came to accept this, she stated, "I responded normally to an abnormal situation."

Finally, the exorcism makes explicit that demons as symbolic representations for the abuse are partial and confusing and need to be renounced and replaced with verbalizable memory. Because the demon allowed for a partial introjection of the sadistic aggression while avoiding the painful remembering of the abuse, the exorcism of this demon, identified as antagonistic to memory, allowed Barbara to go on to the painful abreaction of her sadistic experiences.

An additional advantage of the exorcism paradigm is that it employs the language of the primary process thinking operative within the child at the time of the original trauma. Memory of a traumatic event is often experienced and reported at the cognitive level of the individual at the time the event occurred. Fairbairn (1927/1954a) has noted that religious language is quite close to the primary process. When the exorcist uses the language of demonic and divine entities residing within her and commands the demons to leave, he enters the world of the patient's childhood experience and meets her with what she feels to be powerful and empathic assistance. Her anxiety level is reduced, and this frees her secondary process skills for later use in integrating the experience and bringing it to the level of symbolization.

Insofar as the exorcism acted as a "transference cure," fulfilling her fantasy of finding a good father figure, it may have shielded Barbara from fully realizing the severity of her grandparental abuse and remaining scars. However, in another sense, the exorcist's function in meeting basic needs for protection and mirroring has served as a way station to these more painful realizations about her grandfather's near-absolute lack of concern for her and her grandmother's abandonment of her to the abusers. As Barbara became more able to acknowledge her appropriate anger at her grandfather's sadism and at her grandmother's abandonment of her, her self-blame decreased. This has expanded the scope and depth of her verbally recalled traumatic experiences.

Comparison of the Two Cases

These two cases raise basic questions: What is possession? and why does exorcism work well in some cases? The Haizmann case is of interest because the painter's possession has been interpreted in several different ways. Freud (1923/1953) saw the possession as representing projection of the patient's own unacceptable sexual and regressive wishes. Macalpine and Hunter (1956) saw the possession as providing a symbolic representation for the patient's pregenital confusion about gender and longings to reestablish caretaking from both mother and father. In our review of the case, we highlight the presence of multiple symptoms often associated with physical and sexual abuse. These include the painter's dissociative experiences, possible flashbacks, apparent vulnerability to triggers (such as anniversary reactions), pseudoseizures, autonomic disturbances, self-mutilations, melancholia, sleep disturbance, and substance use. The immersion in an imaginary world of internal demonic and angelic figures is itself seen as a dissociative symptom. The preoccupying image of the devil is seen as a disguised representation of the perpetrator—in effect a partial internalization of the sadistic aggressor. The painter's drawings are compared with the fear-filled and overgenitalized drawings by contemporary patients known to have been sexually abused. They are also seen as a manifestation of the characteristic tendency of sexually traumatized patients to make their complaints through nonverbal rather than verbal means in response to internalized injunctions not to tell.

Why Does Exorcism Help?

In all versions of the Haizmann case, there is consensus that part of the improvement after exorcism resulted from his establishing a connection with people who were accepting and nurturing and who listened. Freud (1923/1953) thought the connection with the exorcising priests allowed Haizmann to satisfy his longing to be cared for by a father but without having to sacrifice his own maleness. Macalpine and Hunter (1956) saw the exorcism process as providing a redifferentiation of male and female nurturance and a reconnection with these sources of emotional sustenance.

In our review of the Haizmann case and in parallel material from the contemporary case of Barbara, we found that the possession experience represented a partial identification with a sadistic aggressor and symbolized the attendant confusing gratifications. In the contemporary case, where more data were available, we were able to see the possession experience as to some extent deliberately created by the sadistic abuser to foil detection and heighten victim compliance. We were also able to understand the role of possession imagery in defending the victim against traumatic memories by providing a pseudoexplanation for symptoms and distress.

In those cases where exorcism relieves symptoms, it is probably because the victim has been helped to differentiate untainted self-experiences from partial identifications with sadistic aggressors. Part of the power of exorcism is that it allows the patient to use his or her own primary process images to symbolically rearrange internal narratives (see Chapter 4). Exorcisms, when successful, also seem to have a role in helping the victim understand and accept personal behavior during the sadistic traumatization as a situational, survival-based response rather than as an aspect of the personality that must remain continuous. In addition, exorcism allows unrestrained abreaction of the terror, rage, horror, and hurt that must be suppressed during the sadistic attack if the child is to survive. Positive effects may depend on this abreactive quality of exorcism, in addition to its cognitive assistance in differentiating and integrating aspects of the sadistic experience, together with the provision of a reliable benevolent context in opposition to the malevolent childhood experiences.

A potential negative effect of the exorcism experience is the reification of a pseudoexplanation for internal pain that will continue to block memory and substitute transference cure for a thoroughgoing understanding of the repressed traumatic injuries and their effects on current functioning. However, when carefully managed and conducted in a context of psychodynamic psychotherapy, the exorcism experience can actually enhance the reconstruction process by increasing the patient's sense of internal safety and self-esteem. Especially when the possession experience has functioned to maintain the sadistic abusers' demands for silence and compliance, questioning the demons' right to remain within the self can give the patient permission to speak out or to express the remembered pain in art, as may have occurred in the Haizmann case.

References

Allison RB: The possession syndrome: myth, magic and multiplicity. Paper presented to the 2nd Pacific Conference of Psychiatry, May 12–16, 1980, Manila, Philippines

Benecke G: Germany in the Thirty Years' War. New York, Edward Arnold, 1978

Brecht B: Mother Courage and Her Children. New York, Pantheon, 1970

Cockburn JS: Crime in England, 1550–1800. Princeton, NJ, Princeton University Press, 1977

Davis W: Dojo: Magic and Exorcism in Modern Japan. Stanford, CA, Stanford University Press, 1980

Demos JP: Entertaining Satan: Witchcraft and the Culture of Early New England. New York, Oxford University Press, 1982

Ergang R: The Myth of the All-Destructive Fury of the Thirty Years' War. Pocono Pines, PA, Craftsman, 1956

Evans H: Harlots, Whores and Hookers: A History of Prostitution. New York, Taplinger, 1979

Evans RJW: The Making of the Habsburg Monarchy 1550–1700. Oxford, Clarendon Press, 1979

Fairbairn WRD: Notes on the religious phantasies of a female patient (1927), in An Object-Relations Theory of Personality. New York, Basic Books, 1954a, pp 183–196

Fairbairn WRD: The repression and the return of bad objects (with special reference to the war neuroses) (1943), in An Object-Relations Theory of Personality. New York, Basic Books, 1954b, pp 59–81

Freud A: The Ego and the Mechanisms of Defense. New York, International Universities Press, 1966

Freud S: A Seventeenth Century Demonological Neurosis (1923), in The Standard Edition of the Complete Works of Sigmund Freud, Vol 19. Translated and edited by Strachey J. London, Hogarth Press, 1953, pp 69–105

Freud S: Letters to Fliess No. 56 and 57, January 17 and 24, 1897, in The Origins of Psycho-Analysis: Letters to Wilhelm Fliess, Drafts and Notes, 1887–1902. Edited by Bonaparte M, Freud A, Kris E. New York, Basic Books, 1954, pp 187–192

Goodman FD: How About Demons? Possession and Exorcism in the Modern World. Bloomington, IN, Indiana University Press, 1988

Goodwin J: Childhood sexual abuse in psychogenic non-epileptic seizures, in The Dilemma of Non-Epileptic Seizures. Edited by Rowan AJ. New York, Butterworth Heineman (in press)

Grimmelshausen HJC von: Courage, the Adventuress (1670). Translated by Speier H. Princeton, NJ, Princeton University Press, 1964

Grimmelshausen HJC von: Simplicissimus (1668). Translated by Goodrich S. New York, Hippocrene, 1989

Hill S, Goodwin JM: Satanism: Similarities between patient accounts and pre-Inquisition historical sources. Dissociation 2:39–44, 1989

Macalpine I, Hunter RA: Schizophrenia: 1677. London, William Dawson and Sons, 1956

Marshburn JH: Murder and Witchcraft in England, 1550–1640. Norman, OK, University of Oklahoma Press, 1971

Parker G: The Thirty Years' War. Boston, MA, Routledge & Kegan Paul, 1984

Saxena S, Prasad KVSR: DSM-III subclassification of dissociative disorders applied to psychiatric outpatients in India. Am J Psychiatry 146:261–262, 1989

Steinberg SH: The Thirty Years' War and the Conflict for European Hegemony 1600–1660. New York, WW Norton, 1967

Trevor-Roper HR: The Crises of the Seventeenth Century. New York, Harper & Row, 1968

Walker DP: Unclean Spirits. Philadelphia, PA, University of Pennsylvania Press, 1981

Wedgwood CV: The Thirty Years' War. London, Jonathon Cape, 1938

Chapter 4

Possession and Persecution by Demons: Janet's Use of Hypnotic Techniques in Treating Hysterical Psychosis

Eliezer Witztum, M.D.
Onno van der Hart, Ph.D.

When a person believes him- or herself to be possessed or persecuted by a demon, this can be described as a possession syndrome. Another description would be hysterical psychosis (HP). Some authors would even argue in favor of a diagnosis of multiple personality disorder (MPD). All three diagnostic categories are trauma induced and have dissociative features. It is possible that they are functionally equivalent, differing in their clinical picture according to types and patterns of trauma, cultural background of the patient, and explanatory models used by the clinician (Bourguignon 1979; Kenny 1981; Krippner 1987; Varma et al. 1981). The following cases focus on the diagnostic categories of HP and possession syndrome.

We will describe two patients who were diagnosed with HP by their clinicians: Achille, Pierre Janet's patient a century ago in France, who believed he was possessed by the devil, and Avraham, a patient we treated in Israel a few years ago. In both cases, HP could be seen as a posttraumatic stress response characterized by dissociative features.

In this chapter, we focus on the cultural, symbolic, and dissociative nature of trauma-induced HP and its treatment using hypnosis. We review the early and more recent literature on HP, emphasizing Janet's dissociation model, and we identify cultural factors influencing the patient's and clinician's choice between a diagnosis of HP or of possession syndrome. Given the dissociative nature of HP, we advocate psychotherapy using hypnosis as the treatment of choice rather than drug therapy. Both Janet's case study of a century ago and our case example demonstrate the efficacy of hypnosis.

Hysterical Psychosis

The concept of hysterical psychosis (HP) has suffered a curious fate in the history of psychiatry. During the latter half of the nineteenth century, this disorder was well known and thoroughly studied, particularly in French psychiatry. In the early 20th century, the diagnoses of hysteria and of HP fell into disuse. Patients formerly thought to have HP were rediagnosed as having schizophrenia or as being malingerers. Clinicians have subsequently attempted to reintroduce the diagnostic category of HP, but it has not regained official recognition. The Index of the DSM-III-R (American Psychiatric Association 1987) contains HP, then refers readers to either Brief Reactive Psychosis or to Factitious Disorder with psychological symptoms. Brief Reactive Psychosis, first included in the DSM-II (American Psychiatric Association 1968), was considered a response to major stress, such as the loss of a loved one or the psychological trauma of combat.

Early Literature on Hysterical Psychosis

Moreau de Tours (1845/1973, 1855, 1865, 1869) distinguished two modes of mental life: life in the external world and life in dreams. The modes are separated from each other by sleep. The psychotic individual "dreams while awake." The psychosis is a continuation of a dream in the waking state (Moreau de Tours 1855). In chronic psychosis, patients are completely absorbed in their internally generated worlds. They have jumped into a dream state from which nothing can pull them out. According to Moreau de Tours (1865, 1869), HP was a brief and often intermittently recurring psychosis in patients with hysteria.

Hysteria was not well defined at that time, but one of its characteristics was thought to be somnambulism. Moreau de Tours (1865, 1869) and some of his contemporaries found four basic features of HP: 1) its similarity to dreams, 2) its curability (using psychotherapy), 3) its plasticity or polymorphism, and 4) its analogy with chemically induced (as by hashish) "artificial delirium."

Hysterical Psychosis in Janet's Dissociation Theory

Pierre Janet, the most important French authority on hysteria and HP, viewed HP in much the same way as Moreau de Tours (Janet 1894/1898a, 1911b). Janet emphasized that HP constitutes a kind of waking dream in which the subject gradually loses the ability to differentiate between dream elements and normal perceptions. In hysterical attacks, in ecstasies, and in somnambulism, patients play or speak out their dreams. These dreams usually take place in abnormal states or subconsciously, and they disturb the normal thought process by diminishing the disposable force of attention. Janet (1894–1895/1898b) said that a psychosis could be considered hysterical if its dissociative nature could be established. The criteria for that are as follows:

1. The psychosis is embedded in dissociative phenomena;
2. The psychosis itself can be seen as a dissociated mental state;
3. Splitting or doubling of the mind (dédoublement de la personnalité) occurs;
4. Subconscious phenomena are present; and
5. Altered states of consciousness occur.

Janet (1889) defined dissociation as the splitting off, separation, and isolation of certain parts of the personality from the conscious awareness and control of one's habitual personality. These split-off parts of the personality remain unknown to waking consciousness and start to lead lives of their own. They alternate with the habitual personality in dominating the patient's behavior (Van der Hart and Horst 1989). Through clinical observation of many hysterical patients, Janet established that these dissociations were in many cases related to traumatic experiences (Janet 1889, 1898c, 1911b; van der Kolk and van der Hart 1989). The extreme emotions (e.g., anxiety and panic) experienced during the trauma trigger dissociative reactions.

The simplest and most basic forms of dissociated phenomena, memories of traumatic experiences, were labeled as "primary idées fixes" or primary emotional states (Janet 1894/1898a, 1898c). Dreams and fantasies based on these traumatic memories are "secondary idées fixes" or secondary emotional states. The most complex are the alter personalities of patients with MPD, each of which has its own identity and distinguishes itself from the habitual personality.

As we understand Janet, the subject experiences HP as a waking dream based on a traumatic experience (Janet 1894/1898a, 1898c). The subject presents as if in a delusional state that has no apparent connection to his or her current reality. Janet emphasized the fact that the dissociative nature of hysteria implies high hypnotizability. Hypnotherapy was the treatment of choice in these cases (van der Hart et al. 1989).

The early views of Breuer and Freud (1893–1895/1955a, 1893–1895/1955b) on hysteria and HP were strongly influenced by Janet, as Breuer testified (see Chapter 7). They emphasized, among other things, the traumatic origins of these disorders. Breuer also pointed to the dreamlike nature of HP and to the often rapid alternation of such dreams with the normal waking state. He believed that patients dreaming these waking dreams were in a state of self-hypnosis—what the French termed "somnambulism." Unlike Freud, Breuer believed that such "psychotic states" could persist for a long time, as exemplified by the case of Anna O.

The Decline of Hysteria

At the beginning of the 20th century, interest in HP, hysteria, and hypnosis had vanished. The few attempts to establish the clinical validity of HP were not accepted. This led to regarding patients suffering from HP and MPD as malingerers or as following suggestions. Furthermore, Bleuler's introduction of the term "schizophrenia" (Bleuler 1911/1950) as a diagnostic entity encompassing widely divergent mental disorders may have led to the decline of diagnostic entities such as MPD or HP (Maleval 1981; Rosenbaum 1980). Bleuler opposed strongly the diagnosis of HP:

> I have never yet had any reason for making a diagnosis of "hysterical psychosis." All cases so diagnosed by others differed in no wise from other schizophrenics. When a supposed hysteric becomes psychotic or deteriorates, he is in my experience not a hysteric at all but a schizophrenic. (Bleuler 1911/1950, p. 289)

Bleuler's influence was so great that after 1911, the majority of psychiatrists, including Freud, no longer used the diagnosis of HP (Maleval 1981).

The careful clinical studies of Janet and others, which had proved that hysteria and HP are distinct clinical entities with dissociation as the essential feature, were overlooked. Both syndromes required a special treatment approach—namely, psychotherapy using hypnosis, which was used by very few clinicians (Breukink 1923, 1924, 1925). Most clinicians struggled with treating cases of hysteria or HP that were formally diagnosed as "schizophrenia" but that did not neatly fit the diagnostic criteria of schizophrenia.

Dissociation Rediscovered

After World War II, several attempts were made to revive the concept of HP. In line with Janet's dissociation model, the Dutch psychiatrist Hugenholz (1946) stated that HP can develop in individuals with hysterical characteristics who are exposed to traumatic events. These events evoke and reactivate dissociated earlier painful experiences with their associated affect, such as resentment and hate. Patients with HP exhibit a lowering of consciousness, dreaming, fantasizing, staring, inattentiveness, and abulia (loss of will power); the disorder can be complicated by other hysterical symptoms such as abasia (inability to walk), astasia (incoordination with inability to stand), and aphonia.

In America, the work of Hollender and Hirsch during the 1960s became influential. To these researchers, HP is characterized by a sudden and dramatic onset temporally related to a profoundly upsetting event or circumstance and by a short duration (less than 3 weeks). Its manifestations include hallucinations, delusions, depersonalization, and grossly unusual behavior (Hirsch and Hollender 1969; Hollender and Hirsch 1964).

Janet's dissociation model reappeared in the work of Pringuet (1977), who underscored the dissociative aspects of HP, including the doubling of the personality, conversion symptoms, and suggestibility. Spiegel and Fink (1979) stated that HP usually involves brief and intense periods of psychotic behavior, generally with graphic decompensation, severe environmental stress, and rapid recompensation in individuals with other hysterical features. They found that these patients have a poor response to antipsychotic medication but will respond to individual and family therapy. Steingard and Frankel (1985) explicitly stated that dissociation underlies the phenomenon and that certain highly hypnotizable people are prone to experience transient but severe psychotic states while in spontaneously occurring trance. The researchers believed hypnotherapy to be the treatment of choice.

Hysterical Psychosis and Possession Syndrome

Many individuals with HP, including the two patients described in this chapter, experience hallucinations in which possession or persecution by a devil or demon plays a dominant role (Aikins 1929; Spiegel and Fink 1979). In other words, they are in possession states. Similarly, students of possession emphasize its dissociative nature (Zusane and Jones 1989). Comparing HP and possession syndrome, Langness (1976) concluded that they are functionally equivalent. He observed that in cultures where such cases are diagnosed as HP, the diagnosis of possession state is absent, and vice versa.

The important cultural differentiator in this dichotomy is whether the culture is characterized by religious beliefs in spirits. Belief in possession and religious tradition have always gone together. Thus, in Christianity, the Roman Catholic church has always recognized possession by the devil, and exorcists have existed since the third century to treat such cases. In Judaism, the soul of a dead person may enter someone's body during the course of his or her life, not just at conception or birth (Bilu 1985). In Jewish mystical communities adhering to this doctrine, *dybbuk* possession was a well-known phenomenon. In India today, belief in supernatural entities and transmigration of souls is still an important part of the Hindu and Buddhist traditions. In a recent survey of dissociative disorders, records of 2,631 patients seen in adult outpatient services in India were screened for dissociative symptoms (Saxena and Prasad 1989). In 62 cases, a DSM-III (American Psychiatric Association 1980) diagnosis of dissociative disorder could be given; 9.7% of these patients had a possession syndrome (with MPD being conspicuously absent). Clinical observations indicate that possession syndrome is also common in other South Asian countries (Adityanjee et al. 1989).

Not all possession cases are culturally regarded as pathological or demonic. It is important to distinguish between "normative" ritual possession, which serves social functions, and "peripheral possession" (Ward 1980). The latter represents the long-term, pathological reactions with control by malevolent or immature spirits (Krippner 1987; Ward 1980; Zusane and Jones 1989). It is often the patient's local community or sect that interprets his or her behavior as pathological (i.e., as a possession syndrome; Langness 1976).

In conclusion, where possession states are a recognized part of a culture, the community and local clinicians tend to speak of possession syndrome in pathological cases. In dominant Western culture, HP or a related diagnosis (such as MPD) will be used. As Kenny (1981) has shown us, William James (Taylor 1982) was probably the first to recognize this when he ironically remarked, "If there are real demons they might possess only hysterics."

Treatment

Our discussion of the literature on the traumatic origins, dissociative nature, and cultural mode of HP, sometimes characterized as possession state, points to at least three principles that should guide clinicians in their assessment and treatment of patients with this trauma-induced disorder:

1. The dissociative nature of the disorder should be established and treatment should be based on its recognition. This implies psychotherapy using hypnosis as the treatment of choice, with medication having an auxiliary function (Breukink 1923, 1924, 1925; Hoek 1868; Janet 1898c; Spiegel and Fink 1979; Steingard and Frankel 1985; van der Hart and van der Velden 1987). Hypnosis is the most powerful medium for transforming the patient's pathological imagery.
2. The traumatic origins of the disorder should be traced and become the focus at the appropriate stage of treatment (Brown and Fromm 1986; van der Hart et al. 1989).
3. When Western-oriented clinicians treat these patients, they should treat them within the context of cross-cultural therapy. They should allow these patients to articulate and resolve their dissociative symptoms in the mode of the prevailing idiom and metaphors of their unique cultural background (Crapanzano 1975; Good and Good 1986; Witztum et al. 1990).

In the two following case studies, similarities are striking despite vast differences in time and cultural background, which demonstrates how these treatment principles are relevant in widely different contexts.

Case Study 1: Achille—Possession by the "Devil"

Janet (1894–1895/1898b), reports that Achille, 33—elsewhere called Daill (Janet 1893/1911a)—was admitted to the Salpêtrière in a state of HP. He presented with unintelligible speech and actions, reporting that he saw the devil, black and horned, sneering at him. He heard one demon whispering menaces, damnation, and pernicious advice and felt another in his chest forcing him to utter blasphemies.

Achille, though somewhat fearful, had been a cheerful, happily married family man. Although both his parents had been alcoholic and his father had also been very superstitious, Janet pronounced Achille as having had a rather normal childhood. Achille had been a sensitive and assiduous boy who read a great deal. He was highly impressionable, taking everything seriously "as if it all really happened like that." After a punishment or small insult, he could be upset for days. He was unable to make friends, and at school he was often the butt of ridicule. However, his marriage, at age 22, proved developmentally fortunate; his wife was a dedicated woman able to keep him in touch with reality and make a happy man of him. They had a daughter, who developed quite normally. For 12 years, everything went smoothly.

At the end of the winter of 1890, a year before his admission, Achille returned home from a business trip in a sour mood, became extremely uncommunicative, and avoided contact with his wife and daughter. Shortly thereafter, he lost his power of speech. When he regained it, he was extremely anxious and felt he was being choked. Several doctors were consulted who made varying diagnoses of somatic illnesses. Achille stopped eating, became immobile, barely spoke, and avoided all contact with his wife and daughter. One morning, he laughed satanically for hours, terrifying everyone present. Afterwards, he saw and heard demons, felt them within himself, and behaved quite oddly.

Janet viewed this as the exterior (symptomatic) aspect of Achille's illness. He believed there was another state, dissociated from this one, in which the patient could explain his illness clearly. Janet was able to evoke this state by using hypnosis. Direct attempts to hypnotize the wildly gesticulating, ranting man were unsuccessful, preventing a traditional induction. However, while Achille was in the midst of hallucinating, Janet slipped a pencil into his hand, carefully guiding the hand to write the name "Achille." The writing spontaneously turned into automatic writing, which Janet interpreted as originating from a dissociated state. Janet then tried verbal commands. While Achille was still distracted, Janet seated himself behind him and softly suggested that he would make certain movements. The movements were not made, but to Janet's surprise the hand rapidly wrote.

"I don't want to."

"And why don't you want to?" Janet responded softly.

"Because I am stronger than you are."

"Who are you then?"

"I am the devil."

"Oh, very well, then we can talk to each other."

To subject the "devil" to his control, Janet appealed to his weak point, his vanity.

"I don't believe in your power and I won't believe in it unless you give me proof."

"What proof?" asked the "devil."

Janet instructed him to allow the left arm of the patient to rise without the patient knowing it. This was done, and Janet gave a series of instructions of the same sort, all of which were performed by the "devil."

Then Janet demanded a final proof: The "devil" was to hypnotize Achille without his noticing it. This, too, was done. The patient slumped over in a deep trance state. Once hypnotized, Janet addressed Achille and elicited the cause of his present condition: During the business trip at the end of the winter in 1890, he had a brief extramarital affair. Afterwards he was tormented by remorse and by the idea of having caught a contagious disease; this was why he had avoided contact with his wife and daughter. Following the doctors' diagnoses of physical illnesses, he dreamt that he died from illness; it was after this that he became immobile.

Janet remarked, "When one has dreamt that one has died, what is there left to dream about? After death, hell." Thus the dreams about demons who came to torture him in hell. To Janet, it was at this point that the subconscious dream amplified, intruding on the patient's normal consciousness in the form of hallucinations. Achille's belief that he was indeed in hell and possessed by the devil determined the content of his delusional ideas.

Achille's remorse about his sexual misdeed was so intense that he experienced it as traumatizing. This emotional flooding in connection with his immoral behavior was the traumatic root of his disorder. Janet's treatment plan was to detraumatize the emotionally overwhelming event and discharge Achille's remorse. He accomplished this by using his hypnotic substitution technique. "An idea, a memory can be seen as a system of images which one can destroy, by separating its elements, by changing these isolated elements, by substituting in this compound one partial image or another for existing ones" (p. 404). Janet did not go into detail, but remarked that "the memory of his [Achille's] misdoing was transformed in all respects because of suggested hallucinations. Finally Achille's wife herself, evoked by hallucination at the suitable moment, completely forgave this more unfortunate than guilty husband" (p. 404).

Once out of hypnosis, Achille felt very much relieved and liberated. He regained all his memories and began to use critical judgment on his delusions. Within a couple of days he was able to laugh about his devil, explaining the delusion to himself as a result of having read too many novels.

However, the delusion continued to haunt him in his sleep, during nightmares in which devils were torturing him. Traces of the delusion were also discernible in automatic writing. Janet therefore applied his substitution technique again, and these dreams also disappeared. Janet concluded that the "devil" was beaten and had disappeared forever. It became difficult to evoke automatic writing or to induce the deep hypnotic state which Achille had attained in previous stages of treatment. The unity of the mind was reestablished. For Janet, the disappearance of the pathological dream (symbolic reliving of the highly charged emotional experience)—which he called an idée fixe—indicated the resolution of the traumatically induced dissociation. The hysterical psychosis remitted completely.

Follow-up at 3 and 7 years indicated that Achille was doing well in all respects.

Case Study 2: Avraham—Persecuted by a "Demon"

On October 16, 1986, terrorists threw three hand grenades into a crowd near the Western Wall in the Old City of Jerusalem, killing one person and wounding 69. Two months later, Avraham, 35, an ultraorthodox

Israeli Jew, was brought to a mental health outpatient clinic by his wife. During the intake session, Avraham frequently cried and moaned as if in physical pain. His affect was depressed. He was oriented to place and time but not to current events. His cooperation with the therapists was so poor that it was impossible to evaluate him accurately for a thought disorder. He denied suicidal tendencies. A tentative diagnosis of Major Depressive Episode was made, and treatment with an antidepressant medication was initiated.

Avraham, accompanied by his wife, attended therapy weekly. During the first 3 sessions, the following background information was gathered from Avraham's wife, as the subject himself hardly spoke. His father, Avraham's first Torah teacher, was, in his time, a well-known Orthodox rabbi and Kabalist. The father was killed in a car accident when Avraham was 8 years old. His mother never recovered from her grief and was incapable of caring for Avraham and his 8 siblings. At the age of 12, he was placed in an orphanage. He studied in a series of Orthodox yeshivas (religious schools that emphasize Jewish studies to the exclusion of secular subjects). At 20, he married and subsequently had 5 children.

As an observant Jew, Avraham frequently went to the Western Wall, the last remains of the Second Temple, the most sacred site in Judaism. Praying there was a continuation of his father's religious habits. Avraham was thus engaged during the evening when the hand grenades were thrown. He was not hit, but the force of the explosions threw him into the air. As far as he remembered, he had not been unconscious. According to his wife, he immediately returned home.

Over the next 2 weeks, Avraham's wife noted a marked change from his normal behavior. He began talking to himself in fragmentary sentences, speaking constantly of bombs and people dying. He was easily startled and distracted. He paid little attention to the family. During the third week, he began to consume huge quantities of food, even compulsively taking food from his children's plates. Over the next month, he gained more than 15 kilograms, developing peripheral edema and episodes of cellulitis that required medical attention. During the fifth week he withdrew further, had extensive crying spells and was obviously depressed. He experienced severe sleep disturbances, including insomnia and periods of shouting and crying during apparent sleep. He refused to bathe, shave, or change his clothes, completely neglecting personal hygiene and appearance. Because of poor attendance and his inability to concentrate on his studies, Avraham was dismissed from the yeshiva, and the family lost its sole source of income. Apart from his deranged behavior, which led his wife to bring him to the clinic, the family's deteriorating economic situation became a stressful factor of increasing magnitude.

Despite the patient's initial presentation as psychotic, he was not responsive to antipsychotics, which were withdrawn along with antidepressants after 1 month. Because the precipitating event was traumatic and followed by rapid deterioration, Brief Reactive Psychosis was the logical diagnosis. However, Avraham was not responsive to medication, and his symptoms persisted for several weeks. We as therapists began considering another possibility. We noticed severe regressive characteristics: Avraham's behavior resembled that of a frightened child—terrified affect rather than detached or remote behavior. He showed no aggressive tendencies. The content of his "hallucinations" was polymorphic, bizarre, and colorful, but also ambiguous and vague. These features were seen as congruent with diagnosis of posttraumatic stress response with strong dissociative features. As more evidence emerged to support this position, we initiated a treatment plan accordingly.

Avraham's Treatment

Whenever the traumatic event at the Western Wall was mentioned in session, the therapists observed that Avraham made agitated arm movements: first upward and then back and forth horizontally. Following Janet, the therapists regarded these movements as expressions of flashback phenomena, iconic representations of overwhelming experiences during the attack: the explosions and people falling and running into each other in panic. When they inquired about this, the patient, who until then had barely spoken in sessions, cried and moaned and began haltingly to explain what had happened.

During the following sessions, Avraham and his wife explained that his frequent prayers at the Western Wall had a dual nature: both to pray and to show respect for the memory of his late father. The attack shattered Avraham's defenses against the unresolved traumatic grief following his father's untimely death. His subsequent compulsive eating was his effort to fill the deep emptiness he felt at the loss of his father.

The therapists made this unresolved grief the focus of treatment. They asked Avraham to write a leave-taking letter to his father in which he could tell his father everything he wanted and needed to tell him (van der Hart 1983). Avraham's wife assisted him in this task. The letter he brought to the next session began with the words, "Father, father, father, why did you leave me? Why didn't you come when I was married?" The handwriting in the first sentence was appropriate for a 35-year-old man, but it quickly degenerated into a disorganized pattern, with large letters typical of the handwriting of a young child, and by the end it had become a scribble. Avraham was asked to read the letter aloud, and the same regression was noted. Although he began in a composed manner, he soon alternated between episodes of screaming and hitting himself vigorously on the chest, and episodes of sinking into a state of masticatory movements of sucking and rocking back and forth. The traumatized child part of his personality reexperienced the intense grief of the loss of his beloved and powerful father. With deep emotion, he expressed the feeling that he would "forever be alone, that life would never be the same, and that forever there would only be a cloud of emptiness."

After this session, the frequency of his nocturnal persecutory attacks increased and persisted into the day as well. He began to eat even more. The continuing weight gain caused additional medical complications, which often prevented him from attending scheduled therapeutic sessions.

The therapists realized they had to explore the nature of these intrusive nocturnal episodes. These experiences occurred mainly during sleep, in the transition state from sleeping to waking, and finally, during the waking state itself. In them, Avraham was threatened by a bizarre figure whom he initially described as "the Black." Additional information from him and his wife, who kept a diary on these attacks, revealed that this ugly creature was nonhuman and had red eyes and the legs of a chicken, the stereotypical description of a demon in traditional Jewish folk religion. When this vision occurred, Avraham would run around the room shouting for help and hitting his head against the wall, trying vainly to shake off the frightening images. During this period he refused to leave the house and kept all windows and curtains closed, because he believed that people were trying to kill him.

The therapists decided to use hypnosis as a means of entering and controlling these frightening dissociative experiences. The hypnotic state was very easily induced. Avraham was directed to see the black figure who was mocking and threatening him: "I killed your father and now I will kill you like I killed him." Avraham also reported seeing his father standing in the shadows looking at him sadly. He cried to his father for help, but his father could not help him. He tried to escape from the black figure but was unable to do so. He could admit that the figure was a "demon," a courageous admission in light of the cultural taboo against naming demons or discussing them.

In the next sessions, the therapists assisted Avraham in gaining some control over this demon. Under hypnosis he was given the traditional instructions for exorcising a demon. Whenever he saw the black figure, he was to incant loudly and clearly: "Go, go, go away, because you do not belong to our world." He used this incantation in hypnosis during the session and saw "the Black" running away. At home in the presence of his wife this incantation was effective, but when Avraham tried to utter it alone it was not.

In order to promote Avraham's ability to cope with the dream when alone, the therapists instructed him to demand forcefully that the "demon" tell him its name. This derived from traditional beliefs that knowing and identifying a demon by name is a prerequisite for overpowering it. Avraham rehearsed this during the session, but the "demon" refused to disclose its identity and ran away. To generate a greater sense of self-control, the therapists taught Avraham self-hypnotic relaxation techniques to practice at home with his wife's assistance.

During the next session, Avraham reported some improvement after using these techniques. When he, in the company of his wife, demanded that "the Black" reveal its name, the "demon" again became frightened. "The Black" now enlisted two aides, and this demonic triad tried, almost successfully, to drown Avraham when he was in the Miqveh (ritual bath).

Therapy reached a stalemate, as Avraham could not engage the "demon." In order to break through the stalemate in the next session, Avraham was asked to visualize the setting where he had last seen the "demon" and its aides. "A desolate place in the desert," was his reply. The therapists interpreted this as a metaphoric kernel statement (Fernandez 1977) expressing his problematic life situation. The "demon" and its two aides were hidden behind nearby boulders. The therapists urged Avraham to search for signs indicating the direction he should take in order to find protection. At first he saw nothing; then, when encouraged to scan the horizon, he found a distant, small spot of green.

It was suggested that this green spot might be an oasis where he could find shelter, water, food, and the company he was looking for—the latter being an indirect suggestion of symbolically meeting his father. When the therapists suggested that Avraham walk in that direction, the "demon" and its aides immediately appeared, trying to distract him from going his own way. (This symbolized the conflict about separating and becoming independent.) He was asked to demand their names and to lure them toward him, holding them captive until they gave their names. The fact that they were still too afraid to approach him restored some of Avraham's self-confidence. At the end of the session, he was asked how old he felt. "Twelve," he answered; older than before.

Avraham continued his imagery process at home with his wife's assistance. During the next session he was encouraged to advance toward the "green," despite the obstacles and recurrent attacks of the "Black" triad. Avraham and his wife reported that at home, the number of episodes involving the "demon" was greatly reduced. Avraham felt more confident in his ability to control the "demon."

During one therapy session, a demonic aide suddenly appeared, in the form of a black dog, and Avraham repelled it by throwing an imaginary stone. Afterwards, he reported his age as 14.

The "Secret Weapon" and the Regaining of the "Lost Paradise"

During the next session, Avraham reported having found a new and powerful ally in his struggle with the demons: The very famous Tsaddik (righteous man) Rabbi Chaim Ben Attar (1696–1743). Avraham had visited the grave of the Rabbi on the anniversary of his death earlier that week. It is believed that a request made on such a pilgrimage to the grave of a Tsaddik will be granted (Bilu and Abramovich 1985). Avraham visited the grave on the Mount of Olives with many others, but afterwards he remained there alone. He cried, asked for help, and prayed for many hours.

Finally, Avraham felt that his prayers were answered. After that, he felt supported by this Tsaddik and experienced himself as more powerful. This event signified an important shift in the development of an internal locus of control. Without direct instructions from us as therapists, Avraham had initiated action to solve his problem. He began assuming responsibility for his situation and enlisted the help of a wise and powerful father figure, which he internalized.

At home, Avraham worked with his wife to come closer to the green area, determined to reach it during the next session with our help and encouragement.

In the 18th session, Avraham described the green area as a beautiful garden surrounded by a high wall. He circled it and found a gate. Suddenly, "the Black" and its aides tried to grab him and throw him in a pit, but with the power of the Tsaddik and with our encouragement, he showed that the balance of power had definitely changed. He actually shouted to the "demons": "In the name of Rabbi Chaim Ben Attar, I tell you, go away! I am not afraid of you! I am not afraid of you! Go away!" He invoked verses from the Psalms: "He that dwells in the secret place of the Most High shall abide under the shadow of the Almighty . . . " (Psalm 91:1). He stood in the center of the therapy room, actually fighting with his arms and legs, until at last he overcame the "demons" and they withdrew, defeated.

Next, Avraham approached the guardian at the gate, explained that he had to enter the garden, and asked permission to enter. From outside, he saw many beneficent, white-bearded Tsaddikim. Suddenly he saw his father among them, called to him, and asked him to instruct the guardian to let him in. Avraham's affect changed remarkably and his depressed expression completely disappeared as he informed his wife and us that he was entering the Lower Paradise. He said that the air smelled like perfume and that he saw two springs of water. (Avraham's experience of the Lower Paradise was consistent with traditional descriptions of this well-known place in Jewish mysticism.) Encouraged to drink and satisfy his thirst, he described the water as sweet and fresh. He himself appeared completely revitalized.

Then he saw his father again and ran to him, embracing him and talking to him joyfully. He saw his admired grandfather, for whom he was named, and embraced him also. Next he met his own Rabbi who had died in a traffic accident when Avraham was 18. He described these experiences with wonder, excitement, and joy, using Biblical verses to express his feelings. At the end of the session, we suggested that from then on Avraham would have the power of Rabbi Chaim Ben Attar with him, plus the additional protective power of the Tsaddikim and his father, grandfather, and former Rabbi. Internalizing their positive qualities would enable him to be a more functional husband and father. Closing suggestions were given for a comfortable, uninterrupted sleep.

In the next and final session, Avraham's wife brought no notes from home. For the first time in 6 months, there was nothing to report. Avraham was sleeping well at night, and apparently all hallucinations and delusions had disappeared. He felt very good, albeit a bit weak. He had spent considerable time in healthy interaction with his children. Both he and his wife felt that his visit to the Lower Paradise had been a mystic miracle, a great privilege that, traditionally, is granted to only a few very righteous men. Avraham did not want to undergo hypnosis again, as the experience in the Lower Paradise felt completed. During the preceding week, on the anniversary of his father's death, he had visited his father's grave and cried intensely. Afterwards, he felt greatly relieved. (This completed the mourning seen as therapeutically necessary to release the dissociated affect of the first traumatizing event.)

Follow-up

More than 5 years after the terrorist incident, Avraham functions relatively well. He experiences mild sleep problems and is a bit phobic of cars, but evidences no psychotic or paranoid ideation or signs of depression. He goes every day to study at the synagogue and yeshiva.

Discussion

Hysterical Psychosis as a Posttraumatic Stress Response

The immediate cause of HP is usually a traumatic or stressful life event. In addition to environmental stressors, subjective factors can be sufficiently traumatizing to produce a posttraumatic stress response. In the case of Avraham, the environmental stressors, the terrorist attack, and the sudden death of his father at age 8 are widely recognized as extremely upsetting. Avraham's enduring belief that his father abandoned him exemplifies the subjective aspects of his traumatic reaction. An amorous affair, as was the case with Achille, hardly fits the criterion of an event that would be markedly stressful to almost anyone in similar circumstances in that person's culture. With Achille, the conviction of having caught a contagious disease and intense feelings of remorse indicate that sometimes the subjective aspects of such an event are most important.

With Avraham, the trauma of the terrorist attack triggered and activated previous traumatic memories regarding the sudden death of his father and its disturbing aftermath. According to Janet (1903), this gives rise to the phenomenon of "double emotion." The traumatic reaction, characterized by "vehement emotions," relates to both the current trauma and the previous traumatic memories. The person is therefore even more overwhelmed and even less able to make sense of his or her experiences. He or she is more at risk, we believe, to develop a more severe posttraumatic disorder such as HP rather than simple posttraumatic stress disorder (PTSD).

Trauma, Dissociation, and Hysterical Psychosis

Dissociating the experience from normal consciousness is the primary defense against trauma (Janet 1889, 1894/1898b, 1911b; Putnam 1989; Spiegel 1984). Dissociation leads to the formation of mental systems outside the experiencing ego (dédoublement de la personnalité), in Janet's terms. In the cases presented in this chapter, the dissociated traumatic experiences—called primary idées fixes or primary emotional states by Janet—evoked dreams and fantasies—secondary idées fixes or secondary emotional states in which certain highly charged thoughts dominated, giving rise to the supernatural, demonic figures. These contents were borrowed from the internalized cultural-symbolical world of these patients.

Achille was a highly impressionable man living at the end of the 19th century in the French countryside where occasionally possession epidemics still occurred (e.g., in 1860 in the village of Morzine and in 1880 in Verzegnies). His remorse about his amorous affair and his belief in having caught a contagious disease with which he could contaminate his wife and daughter led to his dream and hallucinations in which he died, went to hell as a sinner, and became possessed. Avraham as a child felt abandoned by his revered father, who, in his imagination, could only be killed by a demon. The childhood dream about this demon was reactivated as a posttraumatic reaction to the terrorist attack—first as a nightmare, then a "waking dream" or hallucinations in which he himself had become the target of this demon.

Duration of Hysterical Psychosis

Although it is recognized that PTSD may become chronic, in HP a short duration is regarded as a necessary condition. According to Hollender and Hirsh (1964), HP lasts no longer than 3 weeks; DSM-III-R allows for a duration of 1 month for Brief Reactive Psychosis. The cases of Achille and Avraham, which we consider examples of HP, and other cases (Breukink 1923, 1924, 1925; Hugenholz 1946; van der Hart and van der Velden 1987) support the possibility of a longer duration.

The disturbance resulting from trauma-induced dissociation does not impair the organization of thought processes as does "true" psychotic disorder. As the examples illustrate, even when the patients' behavioral responses do not seem appropriate to the present reality, the patient can narrate the delusional (symbolic) content, comment on it as an observer, and recall and refer to it after experiencing it—all functions that are impaired in psychosis. When their posttraumatic HP episodes are resolved, patients return to their former levels of functioning and thought processing.

Some authors emphasize high hypnotizability in these patients (Breukink 1923, 1924, 1925; Spiegel and Fink 1979; Steingard and Frankel 1985). Both patients described in this chapter showed high trance capacity, although Achille was not easy to hypnotize.

We propose that for a "psychosis" to be HP, its dissociative nature—not its short duration—must be established. According to Janet (1894/1898b), this is apparent in the alteration of different states of consciousness, the presence of subconscious phenomena, and high hypnotizability. This alteration of states of consciousness is referred to in modern literature as the intrusion of traumatic memories, flashbacks, and nightmares. The rapid and persistent intrusion of these traumatic phenomena into daily life creates an alternative reality in which subjects experience themselves. At best, the intrusion is minimal; at worst, traumatic imagery alternates increasingly with current reality until it dominates. It is the subjective experience of this dual reality that defines the psychotic features of HP.

The Role of Hypnosis and Culture-Sensitive Techniques in Treatment

Patients with HP usually respond poorly to antipsychotic medication and have a high degree of hypnotizability. Although systematic research validating these impressions is needed, for the time being they suggest that psychotherapy, particularly with the use of hypnosis, is the treatment of choice.

Hypnosis can be used to diagnose and identify the traumatic experiences that produced this extreme reaction. Thus, Janet identified the nature of Achille's dissociated material and the cause of his psychosis. Using a hypnotic substitution technique, he changed the hallucinations into more positive images, as with Achille's imagined confession of the affair to his wife and her forgiveness of him. Although in this case Janet describes his substitution technique only briefly, contemporary works (Janet 1889, 1894/1898a) show that he used it widely (van der Hart and Horst 1989; van der Hart et al. 1989).

In Avraham's case, relevant information was collected without hypnosis about the traumatic loss of his father and his bizarre behavior after the terrorist incident. The nonhypnotic technique of writing a leave-taking letter (van der Hart 1983, 1988) was used to address the unresolved mourning and caused regression with an intensification of demonic hallucinations. Hypnosis was used, first to explore the nature of the patient's subjective experience of the demon, and subsequently as a means to help the patient defend himself against "the Black." We as therapists introduced traditional counterdemonic measures, such as magic incantations, investigations of the nature of "the Black" and its aides, and demands that it reveal its name and identity.

We then used the hypnotic technique of guided imagery to transform Avraham's metaphoric kernel statement of desolation into a more positive one (van der Hart 1986; Witztum et al. 1988). In this metaphoric imagery, the patient's arduous journey from the desert to the green spot ended in a joyful reunion with his father in the Lower Paradise. This event within the domain of metaphoric imagery, coupled with his visit in real life to the grave of the Tsaddik and the visit to his father's grave, constituted the resolution of his chronic, traumatic grief (Bilu et al. 1990).

Thus, both in hypnosis and in the waking state, we joined and utilized the patient's own language and metaphors, as illustrated in his use of blessings, prayers, and Biblical verses, in order to enter his experiential world and facilitate the healing of his trauma (Good and Good 1986). Instead of trying to convince Avraham of the irrational nature of his hallucinations, we used culture-sensitive therapeutic techniques based on the patient's explanatory model that consisted of traditional religious and mystical sources congruent with his belief system and cultural background.

Conclusion

In this chapter, we have stressed the importance of accurately diagnosing HP or possession syndrome. A recent traumatic event can trigger and combine with past traumata in forming the representational nature of the symptomatology. Hypnotic procedures help therapists enter the patient's world and join and utilize the patient's cultural explanatory model and idiosyncratic symbols to transform this inner world.

We suggest that when a delusional presentation or hallucination follows a traumatic event, the proposed model would prevent the precipitous diagnosis of psychosis and provide an effective treatment approach. This approach is based on our clinical experience and on anecdotal evidence from both historical and recent sources, but more systematic studies are needed.

References

Adityanjee M, Raju G, Khandelwal S: Current status of Multiple Personality Disorder in India. Am J Psychiatry 146:1607–1610, 1989

Aikins H: Casting out a "stuttering devil," in An Outline of Abnormal Psychology. Edited by Murphy G. New York, Modern Library, 1929, pp 175–192

American Psychiatric Association: Diagnostic and Statistical Manual of Mental Disorders, 2nd Edition. Washington, DC, American Psychiatric Association, 1968

American Psychiatric Association: Diagnostic and Statistical Manual of Mental Disorders, 3rd Edition. Washington, DC, American Psychiatric Association, 1980

American Psychiatric Association: Diagnostic and Statistical Manual of Mental Disorders, 3rd Edition, Revised. Washington, DC, American Psychiatric Association, 1987

Bilu Y: The taming of deviants and beyond: an analysis of dybbuk possession and exorcism in Judaism. The Psychoanalytic Study of Society 11:1–32, 1985

Bilu Y, Abramovich H: In search of the Saddiq: visitational dreams among Moroccan Jews in Israel. Psychiatry 38:145–159, 1985

Bilu Y, Witztum E, van der Hart O: Paradise regained: miraculous healing in an Israeli psychiatric clinic. Cult Med Psychiatry 14:105–127, 1990

Bleuler E: Dementia Praecox or the Group of Schizophrenias (1911). New York, International Universities Press, 1950

Bourguignon E: Psychological Anthropology. New York, Holt Rinehart & Wilson, 1979

Breuer J, Freud S: Studies on Hysteria (1893–1895), in The Standard Edition of the Complete Psychological Works of Sigmund Freud, Vol 2. Translated and edited by Strachey J. London, Hogarth Press, 1955a, pp 1–18, 183–252

Breuer J, Freud S: On the psychical mechanism of hysterical phenomena: a preliminary communication (1893–1895), in The Standard Edition of the Complete Psychological Works of Sigmund Freud, Vol 3. Translated and edited by Strachey J. London, Hogarth Press, 1955b, pp 25–42

Breukink H: Over de behandeling van sommige psychosen door middel van een bijzondere vorm der kathartisch-hypnotische methode. Ned Tijdschr Geneeskd 67:1321–1328, 1923

Breukink H: Nadere mededeelingen over de hypnotische behandeling bij sommige geesteszieken. Ned Tijdschr Geneeskd 68:911–918, 1924

Breukink H: Nadere mededeelingen over de behandeling door hypnose bij zenuw-en geesteszieken. Ned Tijdschr Geneeskd 69:1877–1887, 1925

Brown D, Fromm E: Hypnotherapy and Hypnoanalysis. Hillsdale, NJ, Lawrence Erlbaum, 1986

Crapanzano V: Saints, jnun and dreams: an essay in Moroccan ethnopsychology. Psychiatry 38:145–159, 1975

Fernandez JW: The performance of ritual metaphors, in The Social Use of Metaphor: Essays on the Anthropology of Rhetoric. Edited by Sapir J, Crocker J. Philadelphia, PA, University of Pennsylvania Press, 1977, pp 100–131

Good B, Good M: The cultural context of diagnosis and therapy: a view from medical anthropology, in Mental Health Research and Practice in Minority Communities: Development of Culturally Sensitive Training Programs. Edited by Miranda M, Kitano H. Rockville, MD, National Institute of Mental Health, 1986, pp 1–27

Hirsch S, Hollender M: Hysterical psychosis: clarification of a concept. Am J Psychiatry 125:81–87, 1969

Hoek A: Eenvoudige mededelingen aangaande de genezing van eene krankzinnige door het levens-magnetismus. Gravenhage, De Gebroeders van Cleef, 1868

Hollender M, Hirsch S: Hysterical psychosis. Am J Psychiatry 120:1066–1074, 1964

Hugenholz P: Kliniek der psychogene psychosen, in Anthropologische psychiatrie. Deel II: Randpsychosen. Edited by van der Horst L. Amsterdam, Van Holkema and Warendorf, 1946, pp 415–478

Janet P: L'Automatisme psychologique. Paris, Félix Alcan, 1889

Janet P: Histoire d'une idée fixe. Revue Philosophique 37:121–168, 1894. Also in Janet P: Névroses et idées fixes, Vol 1. Paris, Félix Alcan, 1898a

Janet P: Un cas de possession et l'exorcisme moderne. Bulletin de l'Université de Lyon, Dec. 1894–Jan. 1895, pp 41–57. Also in Janet P: Névroses et idées fixes, Vol 1. Paris, Félix Alcan, 1898b

Janet P: Névroses et idées fixes, Vol 1. Paris, Félix Alcan, 1898c

Janet P: Les obsessions et la psychasthénie, Vols 1, 2. Paris, Félix Alcan, 1903

Janet P: Contribution à l'étude des accidents mentaux chez les hystériques. Thêse médicale. Paris, Rueff and Cie, 1893. Also in Janet P: L'État mental des hystériques, 2nd Edition. Paris, Félix Alcan, 1911a

Janet P: L'État mental des hystériques, 2nd Edition. Paris, Félix Alcan, 1911b

Kenny MG: Multiple personality and spirit possession. Psychiatry 44:337–358, 1981

Krippner S: Cross-cultural approaches to multiple personality disorder: practices in Brazilian spiritism. Ethos 15:273–295, 1987

Langness I: Hysterical psychoses and possessions, in Culture-Bound Syndromes, Ethnopsychiatry, and Alternate Therapies. Edited by Lebra W. Honolulu, HI, University Press of Hawaii, 1976, pp 56–67

Maleval J: Folies hystériques et psychoses dissociatives. Paris, Payot, 1981

Moreau de Tours J: Du hachisch et de l'aliénation mentale (1845). Paris, Librairie de Fortin, Masson et Cie. English edition: Hashish and Mental Illness. New York, Raven, 1973

Moreau de Tours J: De l'identité de l'état de rêve et de la folie. Annales Médico-Psychologiques (3e serie) I:361–408, 1855

Moreau de Tours J: De la folie hystérique et de quelques phénomènes nerveux propres à l'hystérie convulsive, à l'hystéro-épilepsie et à l'épilepsie. Paris, Masson, 1865

Moreau de Tours J: Traité pratique de la folie névropathique (vulgo hystérique). Paris, Germer Baillière, 1869

Pringuet G: A propos d'un cas de psychose hystérique. La Nouvelle Presse Médicale 6:441–443, 1977

Putnam F: Pierre Janet and modern views of dissociation. Journal of Traumatic Stress 2:413–429, 1989

Rosenbaum M: The role of the term schizophrenia in the decline of diagnosis of multiple personality. Arch Gen Psychiatry 37:1383–1385, 1980

Saxena S, Prasad K: DSM-III subclassification of dissociative disorders applied to psychiatric outpatients in India. Am J Psychiatry 146:261–262, 1989

Spiegel D: Multiple personality as a post-traumatic stress disorder. Psychiatr Clin North Am 7:101–110, 1984

Spiegel D, Fink R: Hysterical psychosis and hypnotizability. Am J Psychiatry 136:777–781, 1979

Steingard S, Frankel F: Dissociation and psychotic symptoms. Am J Psychiatry 142:953–955, 1985

Taylor E: William James on Exceptional Mental States. The 1896 Lowell Lectures. New York, Scribner's, 1982, pp 93–112

van der Hart O: Ritual in Psychotherapy. New York, Irvington, 1983

van der Hart O: Metaphoric and symbolic imagery in the hypnotic treatment of an urge to wander. Aust J Clin Exp Hypn 13:83–95, 1986

van der Hart O: Coping With Loss: The Therapeutic Use of Leave-Taking Rituals. New York, Irvington, 1988

van der Hart O, Horst R: The dissociation theory of Pierre Janet. Journal of Traumatic Stress 2:397–412, 1989

van der Hart O, van der Velden K: The hypnotherapy of Dr. Andries Hoek: uncovering hypnotherapy before Janet, Breuer, and Freud. Am J Clin Hypn 29:264–271, 1987

van der Hart O, Brown P, van der Kolk B: Pierre Janet's treatment of posttraumatic stress. Journal of Traumatic Stress 2:379–395, 1989

van der Kolk B, van der Hart O: Pierre Janet and the breakdown of adaptation in psychological trauma. Am J Psychiatry 146:1530–1539, 1989

Varma V, Bouri M, Wig N: Multiple Personality in India: comparison with hysterical possession state. Am J Psychother 35:113–120, 1981

Ward C: Spirit possession and mental health: a psycho-anthropological perspective. Human Relations 33:149–163, 1980

Witztum E, van der Hart O, Friedman B: The use of metaphor in psychotherapy. Journal of Contemporary Psychotherapy 18:270–290, 1988

Witztum E, Buchbinder J, van der Hart O: Summoning a punishing angel: treatment of a depressed patient with dissociative features. Bull Menninger Clin 54:524–537, 1990

Zusane L, Jones WH: Anomalistic Psychology: A Study of Magical Thinking. Hillsdale, NJ, Lawrence Erlbaum, 1989, pp 94–96

Section III

Rediscovering Sadism

> Evil is unspectacular
> and always human
> And shares our bed
> and eats at our own table.
>
> W. H. Auden, *Collected Poems*

> One must always go back to de Sade, that is to say, to the natural man, in order to explain evil.
>
> Charles Baudelaire, *Intimate Journal*

> The Black Mass is all nonsense, of course . . . but nonsense, after all, does exist. And minds can get drunk with nonsense.
>
> Charles Williams, *War in Heaven*

> Get into the habit, and there's an end to qualms and regrets; whereas one crime may perhaps leave us uneasy, ten, twenty crimes do not.
>
> de Sade, *Justine*

Editor's Introduction

Pediatrics and psychiatry rediscovered child abuse in the second half of the twentieth century. This discovery has been reluctant and halting, meeting resistance at every step. First, Kempe and colleagues (1962) discovered child battering. Prior to this, it had been thought that infants who presented with bruises, bleeding around the brain, and multiple bone fractures might be suffering from a genetic syndrome. A generation later, just as battering began to be integrated as a possible diagnosis, a few physicians began writing about the sexual abuse of children as if it were a real event that actually took place in some families (Goodwin et al. 1979; Herman 1982; Meiselman 1978). Before this, incest accounts had been dismissed as Oedipal fantasy, and physical signs of incest had been explained variously as related to victim promiscuity; congenital problems, such as absence of the hymen; or the consequences of excessive masturbation. In the last few years, a new syndrome began to be described—sadistic abuse of children (Braun 1990; Burgess 1984; Finkelhor et al. 1988; Hill and Goodwin 1989). Once again, descriptions by children and psychiatric patients were ascribed to fantasy and mass hysteria (Ganaway 1989) and compared to accounts of visits by flying saucers.

As each of these abuse syndromes has been rediscovered, physicians have been surprised to learn that their skepticism had bypassed centuries of folklore, biography, and literature that describe each of these conditions in great clinical detail. "Hansel and Gretel" tells as much as any clinical study about the emotional violence and lies that accompany parental neglect of children. One can go to the lives of Chekhov, Dickens, or Kipling for glosses on this tale and for lifelong follow-up of sequelae (Shengold 1989). The fairy tale "Thousandfurs" and its variants describe the incestuous abuse of children (Goodwin 1989). For modern examples of incest's most serious outcomes one finds many (too many) victim fatalities among notable women in this century, including Virginia Woolf, Marilyn Monroe, and Ann Sexton (De Salvo 1989).

For a literary and biographical guidebook to sadistic abuse, one requires only de Sade, who in the late eighteenth century catalogued its antecedents, varieties, and consequences. Earlier extensive accounts exist as well. Suetonius (1979) described in exhaustive detail the sadistic practices of Caligula and Nero. In the fifteenth century, Gilles de Rais, one of Joan of Arc's captains, confessed his sadistic crimes to the Inquisition, telling how he and his friends would hunt down little boys on horseback and keep them captive in his castle, where the children were tortured, strangled, sodomized, and finally beheaded. The remains of 200 bodies were found. De Sade claimed Gilles de Rais as a role model (Bloch 1948). The fairy tale "Bluebeard" is an expurgated version of this historical episode (Opie and Opie 1974). Skeptics of course say that Caligula and Gilles de Rais were simply the victims of bad publicity and that writers who tell such tales cannot be trusted. I sometimes fantasize a debate at a psychiatric meeting on the question: *Resolved, that no human being in the history of the world has ever intentionally or seriously hurt another.* I would be willing to try to debate the negative but would be resigned to losing.

Why are we so resistant to rediscovering sadism? One answer is that for physicians, sadism hits too close to home. Physicians, like soldiers and policemen, are given social permission to inflict pain under well-defined, well-controlled conditions. We go to great lengths to distance what we must do as physicians from the things sadists do, even developing an elaborate private vocabulary that provides us with substitute words for the pain we must inflict. Physicians do not cut or dismember or mutilate or tie down. We make incisions, perform amputations, and use restraints. We cringe when we discover that our techniques or instruments are used by lay sadists, as when de Sade used medication to poison prostitutes or when he describes amputations as accompaniments to rape. When a physician or nurse begins to practice sadism, as Mengele did at Auschwitz, the practitioner's specialized knowledge and ability to command trust can lead to monstrous violations (Lifton 1986).

When Stoller (1987) searched for prior sadistic victimization in a sample of consensual sadists, he found that more than half had experienced massive medical intervention before age 6. Perhaps it is too much to expect of a very young child to master the fine distinctions between sadism and what physicians do to him or her (see Chapter 9), just as it may be too much to expect of the young child who has survived a riot or been sent to a refugee camp to understand that these acts were not designed in particular to cause pain to him or her (see Chapter 6).

This is why the rediscovery of sadism requires of physicians an especially radical self-examination. No wonder physicians find so many good reasons not to get involved either with sadists or their victims. By and large, we tend to find the victims too ill to treat—mistrustful, delusional, hallucinated, and self-destructive (Goodwin 1988). We find the sadists too healthy; extensive psychological testing of Nazi war criminals yielded normal profiles (Harrower 1976).

Yet there is a sense that these abusers who leave so many explosive fragments of themselves in their victims and in all of us represent a kind of last frontier—a final challenge to those of us who dream of living in freedom, without violence or lies. Perhaps this is part of the enduring fascination of the Marquis de Sade.

References

Bloch I: Marquis de Sade: His Life and Works. New York, Brittany Press, 1948

Braun B: Dissociative disorders as a sequel to incest, in Incest-Related Syndromes of Adult Psychopathology. Edited by Kluft RP. Washington, DC, American Psychiatric Press, 1990, pp 227–246

Burgess AW: Child Pornography and Sex Rings. Lexington, MA, Health, 1984

De Salvo L: Virginia Woolf: The Impact of Childhood Sexual Abuse on Her Life and Work. New York, Ballantine, 1989

Finkelhor D, Williams LM, Burns N: Nursery Crimes. Newbury Park, CA, Sage, 1988

Ganaway GK: Historical truth versus narrative truth. Dissociation 2:205–220, 1989

Goodwin J: The language and politics of caretaking. Pilgrimage 14:10–12, 1988

Goodwin J: Sexual Abuse: Incest Victims and Their Families. Chicago, IL, Mosby Yearbook, 1989

Goodwin J, Sahd D, Rada RT: Incest hoax: false accusations, false denials. Bull Am Acad Psychiatry Law 6:269–276, 1979

Harrower M: Rorshach records of the Nazi war criminals: an experimental study after 30 years. J Pers Assess 40:341–351, 1976

Herman J: Father-Daughter Incest. Cambridge, MA, Harvard University Press, 1982

Hill S, Goodwin J: Satanism: similarities between patient accounts and pre-Inquisition historical sources. Dissociation 2:39–44, 1989

Kempe CH, Silverman FN, Steele BF: The battered child syndrome. JAMA 181:17–24, 1962

Lifton RJ: The Nazi Doctors. New York, Basic Books, 1986

Meiselman K: Incest. San Francisco, CA, Jossey-Bass, 1978

Opie I, Opie P: The Classic Fairy Tales. New York, Oxford University Press, 1974

Shengold L: Soul Murder. New York, Basic Books, 1989

Stoller R: Sadomasochism in the perversions. Panel presented at the annual meeting of the American Psychoanalytic Association, New York, May 1987

Suetonius: The Twelve Caesars. Translated by Graves R. New York, Penguin, 1979

Chapter 5

Human Vectors of Trauma: Illustrations From the Marquis de Sade

Jean M. Goodwin, M.D., M.P.H.

This chapter proposes the term "sadistic abuse" as a descriptor for those extreme and severe acts of interpersonal violence which in the 1980s came to be described as "ritual abuse." One advantage of returning to this older terminology and associated conceptualizations is that it may clarify some of the credibility issues surrounding "ritual abuse." The life and works of the Marquis de Sade provide an encyclopedic historical framework in which to understand patients' accounts of "ritual abuse." Using the life of de Sade as a blueprint, we can anticipate that such accounts will surface not only in ritual or pseudoreligious contexts but also in extreme family violence, pornography, sadistic crime, and political torture. A recent study of incarcerated sadistic criminals echoes details found not only in the accounts of alleged "ritual abuse" victims, but also in the life and pornographic works of the Marquis de Sade.

The term "ritual abuse" began to appear in the 1980s as a descriptor for extremely severe multimodal child abuse. Such accounts were collected from preschool-age children, often in nursery school settings; one study found sadistic elements in 13% of such cases (Finkelhor et al. 1988; Kelly 1989). Descriptions came also from adolescents and adults with severe psychiatric symptoms, often including multiple personality disorder (Snow and Sorensen 1990; Wood and Hatton 1989; Young et al. 1991). Severity indicators found in these accounts included multiple victims; multiple perpetrators often acting together;

This chapter is based on a paper presented at the Annual Meeting of the American Academy of Psychoanalysis in New Orleans, Louisiana, in May 1991.

multiple types of sexual and violent acts; detailed elaborate planning; and certain hallmark acts of torture, including tying down or locking up, insertion of objects, forced eating of nonfood items, mutilation, and killing, especially of infants and animals (Jones 1991). These emotionally devastating actions were described as occurring in an equally devastating setting of hatred, name-calling, and intrusive overcontrol. In many cases, these acts were linked to satanic or other antiestablishment philosophies taught and practiced in family groups, in adolescent gangs, or in other groups organized around a disturbed charismatic individual. However, similar patterns of severe physical and sexual abuse were also encountered in other contexts: 1) severe family violence, 2) pornography and prostitution rings, 3) sadistic crime, and 4) political torture.

Exploration of severe multimodal abuse has been hedged by controversy, much as were the earlier explorations of child battering and, later, incest. Credibility problems are still commonly encountered, with victim fantasy or delusion cited as potential sources for such extreme allegations. As with battering and incest, the acquisition of clinical research data has tended to resolve substantive credibility issues while raising more complex research questions (van Benschoten 1990).

"Sadistic Abuse" Versus "Ritual Abuse"

This discussion focuses on terminology as one contributor to the credibility problems associated with extreme abuse. Rather than "ritual abuse," "sadistic abuse" is proposed as a descriptor for the severe, multimodal abuse picture with torture described previously.

Several authors have pointed out problems with the term "ritual abuse" (Lanning 1989; Lloyd 1990). One drawback is that, as a new term, it ascribes a quality of novelty to observations about severe multimodal abuse. This is misleading. The historical record provides numerous earlier examples. Nonetheless, the misleading aura of novelty leads to further credibility challenges, such as "Why has no one seen this before?" Questions of epidemic hysteria arise that may be more responsive to this terminologic imprecision than to the actualities of the history of child abuse and torture (de Mause 1974, 1991; Stover and Nightingale 1985).

Another problem with designating these phenomena as "ritual abuse" is that the term focuses on motive, which is always more difficult than actions to observe and classify accurately. Failure to highlight behavior is a particular problem here, because torture is a set of behaviors that particularly eludes our focussed attention. Such extreme and emotionally shocking behavior calls forth normal dissociative mechanisms both in perpetrators and victims (Lifton 1986) and is also carried out in secrecy, with shame, deception, and denial further clouding the behavioral reality.

The term "ritual abuse" not only focuses on the more vague and less urgent area of motive but also implies that the motive must be pseudoreligious, rather than sexual, economic, criminal, political, or interpersonal. Any tendency to omit these other aspects of motivation will limit our capacity to explore fully the complex nature of these actions.

Another problem is that the use of the singular term "ritual abuse" for this cluster of diverse behaviors noted in so many different contexts implies a unity within the phenomena that has yet to be demonstrated. Insofar as unities can be anticipated, it is far too early to assume that they will be found only in the religious-philosophical-spiritual area. Thus, the term itself may distort our search for unitary concepts and make such exploration vulnerable to dismissal as witch-hunting, conspiracy-theorizing, or even intrusion into basic religious freedoms.

In contrast, the term "sadistic abuse" takes us into history rather than implying novelty. The Marquis de Sade was a famous pornographer and sexual criminal of the eighteenth century whose career included the perpetration of family violence, the elaboration of a philosophical rationale for his sexual preferences, and an unsuccessful attempt at becoming a political executioner.

The historicity of de Sade goes beyond his own lifetime and touches on the nineteenth-century origins of the concept "sadism" and that term's connections with early psychiatry and trauma theory. The term "sadism" was first used by Krafft-Ebing (1894/1965) as a descriptor for extreme sexual and physical violence. Krafft-Ebing was a friend and mentor of Freud and was moderator at the scientific session in which Freud first presented his paper "The Etiology of Hysteria" (1896/1958). Freud's paper described severe psychiatric symptoms in patients who had been sexually abused in childhood. "A scientific fairy tale," scoffed Krafft-Ebing (Masson 1984). This comment must have been doubly shattering to Freud, who relied upon Krafft-Ebbing not only as a friend but as someone who, as the world's expert on sadism, might be more likely than the rest of the audience to believe that such actions occurred, that such victims existed, and that those victims might be seriously damaged.

The term "sadistic abuse" grounds us not only in history but also in behavior. De Sade's books provide vivid detailed and encyclopedic descriptions of every variation of the sadistic practices that we now hear recounted by victims of severe multimodal abuse. Insofar as the use of de Sade's name implies motive, that motive is sexual discharge. This was de Sade's preferred explanation for his own behavior, and Krafft-Ebing later accepted and elaborated on this hypothesis (1894/1965). However, de Sade's life story is various enough to allow us to reconstruct a more complex set of motives, including not only sexuality but also philosophy, power, money, fame, politics, and the reenactment of his own painful childhood identifications.

Also, the sexual motivations for these acts may bear some additional emphasis and study. These are the motives to which children especially are likely to be entirely oblivious because of their developmental differences in knowledge of and interest in genital sexuality. For a child, it is very difficult to imagine that a beating is taking place for the purpose of producing ejaculation in the perpetrator; it is much easier to imagine a spiritual or religious reason. Thus, an excess emphasis on the sexual aspect of extreme abuse may be useful at this stage, because this aspect of the behavior is so difficult to grasp and so often denied.

Finally, the term "sadistic abuse" brings us toward a more pluralistic and less monolithic view than does "ritual abuse." Not only were de Sade's motivations numerous and complex, but he also gives an example of how philosophies other than satanism can be used to justify extreme abuse. Also, because of use of the term in psychiatry for more than a century, it opens to us not only de Sade's biography but the biographies of other sadists that had been studied by Krafft-Ebing (1894/1965) and his successors. When skeptics ask us to produce a study of ritual abuse offenders, this is somewhat difficult. Perpetrators of sadistic abuse, on the other hand, have been studied in many contexts. If we understand ritual abuse as simply one of many forms of sadistic abuse, then other, more readily available data bases become relevant, including surveys of sadistic criminals, studies of users of sadomasochistic pornography, studies of war criminals, and descriptions of perpetrators of extreme family violence.

The Life and Crimes of the Marquis de Sade

De Sade was born into the French aristocracy in 1740. His father was often away on diplomatic missions, so de Sade was educated by his father's brother, who was an abbé, an aristocratic priest who was not affiliated with a religious order. This uncle was later imprisoned for "debauchery" (Hayman 1978). Sexual preoccupation first became apparent during de Sade's service in the Seven Years' War from age 17 to 23. A family retainer sent to monitor his alarming gambling debts noted that the youth was constantly to be found in brothels. An arranged marriage to the daughter of the President of the Paris Assembly provided de Sade with the most loyal and willing of his masochistic victims. For a description of these three important men in de Sade's life—his father, his uncle, and his father-in-law—one can go to his first full-length pornographic book, *The One Hundred Twenty Days of Sodom,* where the young libertine is accompanied on his sexual adventures by three more seasoned and repulsive sadists—the Duke, the Bishop, and the President. De Sade once wrote to an aunt: "If I have any regrets, it is that I should have been born into such a family" (Lannig 1971, p. 34).

De Sade's first book was written in the Bastille in 1789. A complex course of events had brought him to that time and place. Scandal had first arisen shortly after his marriage; a prostitute complained that de Sade had taken her into a sort of satanic chapel, had masturbated into a chalice and onto a crucifix, and had threatened her with guns and a sword (Hayman 1978). He was imprisoned again years later when a beggar named Rose Keller who de Sade had picked up on Easter Sunday escaped from the room in which he had incarcerated her. Rose Keller said she had been tied up and beaten with a cat-o'-nine-tails and lightly cut with a knife. Then there was a problem at a brothel, when the staff were poisoned by de Sade's gift of chocolate bonbons spiked with the aphrodisiac Spanish fly. De Sade is said to have frequented such brothels accompanied by his valet, who sodomized him while de Sade was sodomizing the prostitutes.

Worse scandal arose when de Sade carried off his wife's younger sister into Spain. De Sade's new liaison enraged the President and his wife, who had their son-in-law condemned to execution in absentia. The sister-in-law, who was a teenager when she met de Sade and a canoness at a convent when they ran away together, died shortly after this adventure. De Sade returned to his wife, who participated with him in orgies that involved kidnapped teenaged maidservants. The victims' parents complained, leading to still more scandal.

De Sade's relatives arranged with the king (who was said to have taken great pleasure in reading the secret police reports on this case) for de Sade to be incarcerated by "lettre de cachet" in the Bastille (Didier 1976; Lely 1957). By 1789, de Sade was one of only a handful of prisoners in the ancient fortress when mobs began to gather outside its walls. "Storm it, storm it," De Sade is said to have shouted through the bars; "they're killing the prisoners." Because of this incitement, he was transferred to the Lunatic Asylum at Charenton just a few days before his pleas were heeded and the Bastille was stormed. (De Sade's own lonely castle was stormed later on in the revolution, perhaps by the still-outraged families of the young servant girls who had been imprisoned there.) Unfortunately, Madame de Sade had not had time to remove her husband's possessions from the Bastille, including the nearly completed manuscript of *The 120 Days of Sodom.* One of the heroes of the Bastille seized this manuscript among other booty. It stayed in that family's possession for more than 100 years. It was finally discovered and translated by Iwan Bloch (yet another friend of Freud's) and published in Vienna in 1904, just a year before Freud himself published the Dora case. Of course, this publication came much too late for de Sade who for the rest of his life mourned the loss of his manuscript and tried to reconstruct it in all his subsequent novels. Publication came too late, too, for Madame de Sade, who paid for her negligence with many an emotional drubbing, and who prudently separated from de Sade while he was still incarcerated.

The 120 Days of Sodom: Encyclopedia of Ritual Abuse

What was in *The 120 Days of Sodom*? The plot runs as follows (de Sade 1789/1987). Four libertines obtain possession of a remote castle for 4 months. They assemble in it a carefully selected cast of victims: 8 little boys, 8 little girls, the 4 wives (or mistresses) of the libertines (each has sexually abused a daughter to teach her to be "wife" for one of the others), 16 teenage boys called "fuckers," and 4 procuresses who act as storytellers during nightly orgies that involve consumption of large quantities of alcohol.

The victims are intricately controlled and regulated, including their defecation and urination, which must be reserved for the sexual uses of the libertines. Costumes are designed for the children, who must also go to school with one of the prostitutes to learn how most gratifyingly to masturbate their masters. A detailed calendar of escalation is designed with dates set for the defloration of each one of the children's orifices. The discipline of the calendar is frequently disobeyed (Gallop 1990). The storytelling by the procuresses is arranged to keep pace with this sexual timetable. For the first month, the stories are to detail the "simple passions"; the "complex passions" are to occupy the second month, then "the criminal passions" and finally "the murderous passions." During the telling of these last stories, almost all of the victims are killed, beginning with the wives.

What passions are detailed in story and deed? To mention a few: locking in cages, threatening with death, burying in coffins, holding under water, threatening with weapons, drugging and bleeding, tying upside down and burning, wearing of robes and costumes, staging of mock marriages, defecating and urinating on victims, killing of animals, having victims witness torture, having them witness homicides, pouring or drinking blood, and taking victims to churches and cemeteries. I mention these acts in particular, because these are 15 of the 16 types of allegations found characteristically in children and adult psychiatric patients complaining of "ritual abuse" in the 1980s and 1990s (Finkelhor et al. 1988; Hudson 1989; Snow and Sorensen 1990; Young et al. 1991). The only one missing from de Sade's (1789/1987) inventory is photography. Clearly, its absence is due simply to lack of technology; its place is taken by use of peepholes and use of stages at the orgies, where each libertine could be seen to perform with his entourage of victims.

Rereading de Sade challenges many of the "credibility problems" raised in the modern-day preschool cases in which allegations of sadistic abuse have emerged. Our society found it incredible that so many different perverse practices were reported by children in these cases. Sixteen types of perversions were, for us, too many. Our prevailing concept of sexual perversion involved the idea that sexual interests and partners would be narrowed in sexual disorders—perhaps to a unitary type of object choice and sexual practice, as seen in certain types of pedophilia. However, this is not the case in sadism. If 16 types of perversions seems a great many, consider de Sade, who describes 600 different perverse practices in *The 120 Days of Sodom* (1789/1987).

"Too many victims," ran another credibility argument in the preschool sadistic abuse cases. "How could so many children have been victimized?" De Sade provides a blueprint in *The 120 Days* for victimizing 32 children. He also describes weekly orgies that the libertines would arrange in town. Procuresses would invite 100 prostitutes; "only too often something less than the full hundred would leave" (de Sade 1789/1987, p. 196).

Still another credibility question involved skepticism that more than one sadistic perpetrator could act successfully in concert. De Sade gives a picture of how and why this is done. Sadists are addicted to these activities; their sexual discharge is profoundly dependent on being seen by each other, cleverly designing and ruthlessly executing sadistic acts. They plan together; anticipate together; are sexually kindled by each other's excitement, erection, or ejaculation; and boast to each other afterward. They are assisted by paid professionals acting from financial as well as sexual and power motives.

Other credibility questions in the preschool sadistic abuse cases concerned the elaborate nature of the arrangements, with minute attention to details of costume and sequencing. "Nobody would go to that much trouble," we were told. It did not seem functional. Why make rape so complicated? However, it is precisely this excess of planning and violence that make the accounts credible as describing sadism. The sadist derives pleasure from the shocked, pained, or confused expression on the victim's face (Heilbrun and Seif 1988). The inflicting of pain and the carrying off of successful deceptions are means to an end, but they are also sadistically gratifying ends in themselves.

Some will say that de Sade is not a reliable informant. He was a pornographer after all, using his own fantasies to pander to the fantasies of others. Can we consider this as evidence that such things are done in reality? We have data that de Sade himself actually practiced some (but not all) of the perverse actions he wrote about.

It seems, for example, that homicidal sadism was an area de Sade explored in fantasy only. After the fall of the Bastille and during the Terror, de Sade threatened to become a darling of the Revolution. Orgies were held in the streets in honor of the goddess of Reason, and de Sade's funeral oration on Marat became the song heard on every street corner (Hayman 1978). De Sade was made a judge in one sector of Paris—as it happened, the very sector where de Sade's hated father-in-law, the President, and his equally hated mother-in-law, were to be tried. De Sade refused to condemn his father-in-law to the guillotine, or anyone else for that matter. He said that, personally, he had never gotten an erection from watching someone be guillotined. Others did, he knew.

De Sade's contemporary Casanova, for example, wrote of the sexual pleasures of seeing a prisoner drawn and quartered (Bloch 1948; Lynch 1984). This was simply not de Sade's cup of tea, although human bones were later found in his castle garden. It is likely, though, that these victims died "accidentally," unable to withstand de Sade's preferred level of torture (Dworkin 1981). Because only sexual motives were allowed in de Sade's philosophy, he refused to do for political reasons something (i.e., guillotining) he would not do for sexual ones. In addition to this dereliction, de Sade faced new regimes that were less charmed by his perversions. So back went de Sade to prison, and eventually to the Lunatic Asylum at Charenton, where the director resumed writing protest letters to the authorities about the inappropriateness of the placement.

Of course, there may have been other reasons for de Sade's refusal to become a political executioner. Lacanian analysts (Crivillé 1990), who view sadism as a displacement of hatred from the father to child and female substitutes, would say that de Sade's entire system would have been threatened catastrophically had he confronted the hated father figure directly.

Despite this well-documented exception, the balance of the evidence leads us to believe that although it is true that some of de Sade's fantasies outran his activities, it is also true that he often fantasized in preparation for action. History teaches that there is no cruelty that human beings have fantasized that we have consistently forborne to enact. A book written a century before de Sade by a priest details tortures identical to some of those in *The 120 Days of Sodom.* However, this book (*A Brief History of the Destruction of the Indies* by las Casas [1552/1974]) is merely history, not pornography, and the victims numbered not in the dozens, but in the tens of thousands.

Research Implications

If we expand the field of inquiry from "ritual abuse" to "sadistic abuse," what clues can we gather that may help us understand the situation of child and adult victims who tell us about extremely severe abuse?

De Sade, like modern-day sadists, elaborated a philosophy to rationalize his sexual crimes. He advocated a combination of radical sexual libertarianism with radical elitism that placed all blame for victimization on the victim. In retrospect, it seems likely that knowledge of this pseudophilosophy would have been helpful in understanding the accounts and symptoms of de Sade's victims. Similar research efforts are under way to understand the pseudophilosophies of modern-day sadists (Goodwin and Dunleavy 1989; Hill and Goodwin 1989).

De Sade was also a pornographer and a patron of prostitutes. Studies of users and producers of sadomasochistic pornography and prostitutes may therefore give us additional insights. For example, surveys of users of S and M magazines (e.g., "Paddles," "Ouch," "Dial-a-Slave," "Stars and Strikes") suggest that these individuals are highly educated and affluent and that most realized their proclivities between ages 14 and 24 (Breslow et al. 1986; Spengler 1977). They have a low tendency to use psychiatry or psychotherapy, and about 20% are entirely dependent on sadomasochistic activity for sexual discharge.

In addition to the above, de Sade was a perpetrator of family violence, battering his wife and sexually abusing his young sister-in-law. Studies of perpetrators of extreme family violence are still few, but case reports indicate the importance of prior criminal history and of psychopathology, including antisocial personality (Smith et al. 1974), paranoia (Goodwin 1989; Schreiber 1973; Schreiber and Arieti 1981), neurologic damage, and alcohol and substance use (Goodwin 1989).

In addition to these activities, de Sade also had a career (albeit a failed one) as a political executioner. Studies of perpetrators of political torture are also limited, with most of the available data describing Nazi war criminals. However, one finds some potential clues here for further research. Studies of Hitler emphasize the role of childhood exposure to violence (Miller 1983), and discussions of Mengele (Lifton 1986) point to the importance of "doubling" and dissociation in torturers. The literature on Hitler also describes an overlapping of multiple sadistic activities as seen in de Sade, with involvements in family violence, pornography and prostitution, drug use, and pseudoreligious rituals, as well as in political torture (Ravenscroft 1973). The many studies on the education of torturers (Suedfeld 1990) concur in the finding that almost all male human beings (females have not yet been adequately studied) can be taught to kill; most can be taught to torture, given a carefully designed training and incentive system. Nadelson (1991) has suggested that the capacity to take pleasure in killing may be an adaptive trait related to our human evolution as hunters and that it may be normally distributed in the population. Nadelson postulates that some postcombat syndromes may include secret and shameful memories of pleasure and even sexual arousal in combat. This theory adds constitutional factors and exposure to killing (this last was a factor in de Sade's case) as possible factors in the development of sadistic behavior patterns.

It is not clear how much overlap exists among these categories of sadists. De Sade may have been somewhat unique in uniting the spheres of sadistic pseudophilosophy, sadomasochistic pornography and prostitution, family violence, and political torture. However, there is evidence that some modern sadists, like Charles Manson, are multiply motivated by involvements in pseudophilosophies, organized crime, and sexual and personal psychopathology (Terry 1987). It is likely there are also participants in each of these categories who never enter any other sphere and who never commit actual crimes. However, De Sade committed some crimes in the eyes of his contemporaries, thus opening for our scrutiny the literature on sadistic criminals.

The Criminal Sadist

Dietz and colleagues (1990) published data on a series of 30 criminals incarcerated for acts judged to have been the result of sexually sadistic violence. The researchers used criteria for sadism very similar to the criteria for severe child abuse mentioned at the beginning of this chapter. They were looking for quantitative excesses of violence, and for certain particular hallmarks such as bondage, imprisonment, and torture.

Once identified, what were these offenders like? All 30 were male; all but one were white. The most frequent other single characteristic in the group (83%; $n = 25$) was that they were collectors—of pornography, guns, trophies taken from victims, police paraphernalia, or detective magazines. Drug abuse, the next most frequent shared characteristic, was present in 50% ($n = 15$).

Dietz and colleagues (1990) found that a personal history of childhood abuse was rarely reported in this population (20%, sexual abuse

[$n = 6$]; 23%, physical abuse [$n = 7$]). However, extensive interviewing and use of collateral data may be necessary to establish the reality of the childhood histories. Forty-seven percent ($n = 14$) acknowledged parental infidelity or divorce as a childhood factor. Prior arrests and prior homosexual experience were each present respectively in 43% of the subjects ($n = 13$). Educational level was fairly high, with 43% ($n = 13$) educated beyond high school. Forty-three percent ($n = 13$) were married, and 33% ($n = 10$) had military experience. Thirty percent ($n = 9$) had impeccable reputations as solid citizens. Excessive driving seemed to be a characteristic of many of them (40%; $n = 12$); this habit often covered their absences during the sadistic crimes. Thirty percent ($n = 9$) had admitted to incest with one of their own children; that amounted to 60% of those subjects who had children.

Characteristics of the offenses committed by the 30 men again provide familiar elements that resonate with our experiences of the severe abuse of children. All offenses involved intentional torture; 93% ($n = 28$) involved careful planning. When one perpetrator was asked how a person might protect him- or herself from sadistic attack, he said that nothing would help, given the constant, careful stalking method the subjects used. Other traits commonly found were binding and gagging of victims (87%; $n = 26$); feeling detached during the events (probably dissociation—87%; $n = 26$); preselected location, sexual bondage, anal rape, and murder (73% each; $n = 22$); and forced fellatio and a variety of sexual acts (67% each; $n = 20$). These are precisely the characteristics found in accounts of ritual abuse and in *The 120 Days of Sodom.*

In view of the difficulty finding bodies to document ritual abuse, it is of interest that concealment of the bodies of victims was admitted by 20 of the 30 offenders (67%) in the incarcerated population (Dietz et al. 1990). Of the known murder victims of these offenders, 28% were discovered in situations where the body was so destroyed by fire, burial, or decomposition that identification of the victim was initially impossible.

Other elements characterizing more than half of the crimes these subjects committed were long periods of captivity (60%; $n = 18$), beating (60%; $n = 18$), vaginal rape (57%; $n = 17$), and serial murders (57%; $n = 17$). Fifty-three percent ($n = 16$) of these offenders recorded the offense in some way (Dietz et al. 1990).

Sexual dysfunction during the event was a factor with 43% of the subjects ($n = 13$). This issue is described graphically in *The 120 Days of Sodom.* The sadist must escalate the amount of torture used in order finally to ejaculate. Keeping a personal item of the victim and being assisted by a partner were characteristic of 37% of the subjects ($n = 11$). These data underscore the prevalence of multiple participants in sadistic offenses, either participating as coperpetrators or as viewers of trophies or photographic records later (Dietz et al. 1990).

How dangerous are these 30 sadistic offenders? Only 22 of the 30 had killed, but those 22 had logged 187 known murder victims (Dietz et al. 1990). Of those who had killed, 5 of the men accounted for 122 of the murders. These numbers underscore the characteristic multiplicity of victims in sadism—a descriptor which, like multiplicity of offenders, is often misconstrued when children complain as a reason not to believe their accounts. Forty-three percent ($n = 13$) of these sadistic offenders had victimized children. Torture techniques included weapons, painful insertion, beating, electric shock, burning, amputation, cutting, and threatening with animals. Two of the 30 offenders admitted to resuscitating dying victims so that they could extend the period of suffering.

These tortures are reminiscent of the self-mutilations seen in ritual abuse victims and encourage us to ask if these symptoms represent reenactments of torture originally done to these patients by others. For example, in the study group that Dietz and colleagues (1990) described, strangling was the preferred method for inflicting torture and death. This observation needs to inform our approach to the differential diagnosis of victims who present with self-choking, with complaints of feeling choked, or with the appearance under stress of erythema around the neck.

I have described the data from Dietz and colleagues (1990) in some detail to illustrate certain traits that occur frequently and are to be expected in the context of sadism, but which, when told by a child or a psychiatric patient to someone naive to these data, might seem fantastic and unbelievable.

De Sade: The Human Dimension

As I mentioned previously, the advantages of the term "sadistic abuse" are numerous. It helps us focus on behaviors rather than on motives. It emphasizes the multiplicity of motives and the importance of the often denied sexual motive. It also acknowledges the multiple settings in which sadistic behaviors occur and invites us to pool research data from various areas in order to further the clinical understanding of victims and perpetrators.

A final advantage of the term "sadistic abuse" is that it gives us a human being to contemplate rather than an abstraction. Victims and therapists often have difficulty seeing the sadist as human. The sadist's extreme moral violations are at a level that risks forfeiture of human status. Also, in his or her grandiosity, the sadist portrays him- or herself as superhuman and beyond ordinary human rules and constraints.

But de Sade seems somehow to have held on to his human status, if only by the skin of his teeth. Even feminist pioneer Simone de Beauvoir (1955/1987) could not help liking him a little. There is humanness in his refusal to guillotine his enemies even if his rationales for forbearance were distorted. It also took some courage and honesty to write as de Sade did about himself and his fantasies, even though he at times also vociferously denied authorship of his works. De Sade even slightly acknowledged the fear behind his assaultive sexuality: "One has to learn to make the best of horror . . . however frightful . . . it ceases to be horrible for you immediately it acquires the power to make you discharge" (de Sade 1789/1987, p. 532). Also, I suspect that de Sade had a hand in the fate that kept him behind bars for 30 years; like Jean Genet (Sartre 1963), he may have known this was the only way to limit the destructiveness of his compulsions. Unfortunately, the amelioration was only relative. There is evidence that de Sade had child sexual victims brought to him even when he was incarcerated at Charenton (Dworkin 1981).

There may be disadvantages to seeing sadism as having a human face. We may be lulled by honey-tongued rationalizers like de Sade into accepting the unacceptable. However, it seems significant that sadists usually do not desire to be seen in this light (i.e., as simply human)—especially not by their victims.

Krafft-Ebing (1894/1965) saw sadism as a universal human trait—one that provides the energy for the painting of gory battle scenes, the performing of painful surgery, the making of the hard decisions of government (such as going to war), and many other necessary human tasks.

Yet, as rational as we can be about "sadism," this rationality often fails us when we deal with "sadists." Freud, who wrote extensively about "sadism" and "sadomasochism," makes only two references in all his works to "sadists" (Guttmann et al. 1980). Both are humorous asides, indicating that the defensive shields and bucklers of humor, so useful to Freud from beginning to end in his career as a champion of honesty, were never more necessary than here.

It is the sadist that victims are coping with—a sadist now internalized and cloaked in the all-powerful colors that he or she prefers. Perhaps if we can begin to describe the sadist's behaviors with greater precision and in simple human proportions, victims can disentangle themselves from these internalized images without relinquishing the universal human energies that fuel the pathological deviations of their victimizers.

References

Bloch I: Marquis de Sade: His Life and Works. New York, Brittany Press, 1948

Breslow N, Evans L, Langley J: Comparisons among heterosexual, bisexual and homosexual male sado-masochists. J Homosex 13:83–107, 1986

Casas B de las: The Devastation of the Indies: A Brief Account (1552). Translated by Briffault H. New York, Seabury Press, 1974

Crivillé A: Child physical and sexual abuse: the roles of sadism and sexuality. Child Abuse Negl 14:121–127, 1990

de Beauvoir S: Must we burn Sade? Translated by Michelson A, in The Marquis de Sade (1955). Compiled and translated by Wainhouse A, Seaver R. New York, Grove Press, 1987

de Mause L: The History of Childhood. New York, Harper Torchbooks, 1974

de Mause L: The universality of incest. Journal of Psychohistory 19:123–164, 1991

de Sade DAF: The One Hundred Twenty Days of Sodom (1789). New York, Grove, 1987

Didier B: The Marquis de Sade. Paris, Derael/Gauthier, 1976

Dietz PE, Hazelwood RR, Warren J: The sexually sadistic criminal and his offenses. Bull Am Acad Psychiatry Law 18:163–178, 1990

Dworkin A: Pornography: Men Possessing Women. New York, Putnam, 1981

Finkelhor D, Williams L, Burns N: Nursery Crimes: Sexual Abuse in Day Care. Newbury Park, CA, Sage, 1988

Freud S: The etiology of hysteria (1896), in the Standard Edition of the Complete Psychological Works of Sigmund Freud, Vol 3. Translated and edited by Strachey J. London, Hogarth Press, 1958, pp 157–185

Gallop J: Thinking Through the Body. New York, Columbia University Press, 1990

Goodwin J: Persecution and grandiosity in incest fathers, in Sexual Abuse: Incest Victims and Their Families. Edited by Goodwin J. Chicago, IL, Mosby-Yearbook, 1989, pp 83–94

Goodwin J, Dunleavy J: What families say: the dialogue of incest, in Sexual Abuse: Incest Victims and Their Families. Edited by Goodwin J. Chicago, IL, Mosby-Yearbook, 1989, pp 65–82

Guttmann S, Jones R, Parrish L: Concordance to the Psychological Works of Sigmund Freud (6 Vols). Boston, MA, GK Hall, 1980

Hayman R: De Sade: A Critical Biography. New York, Crowell, 1978

Heilbrun AB, Seif DT: Erotic value of female distress in sexually explicit photographs. Journal of Sexual Research 24:47–57, 1988

Hill S, Goodwin J: Satanism: similarities between patient accounts and pre-Inquisition historical sources. Dissociation 2:39–44, 1989

Hudson P: Ritual child abuse: a survey of symptoms and allegations. Paper presented at the annual meeting of the International Society for the Study of Multiple Personality and Dissociative Disorders, Chicago, IL, October 1989

Jones DPH: Ritualism and child sexual abuse. Child Abuse Negl 15:163–170, 1991

Kelly S: Stress responses of children to sexual abuse and ritual abuse in day care centers. Journal of Interpersonal Violence 4:502–513, 1989

Krafft-Ebing R von: Psychopathia Sexualis: a Medico Forensic Study (1894). Translated by van den Haag E. New York, Stein & Day, 1965

Lannig W: Portrait of de Sade: An Illustrated Biography. New York, Herder & Herder, 1971

Lanning K: Satanic, occult, ritualistic crime: a law enforcement perspective. Police Chief 56:62–85, 1989

Lely G: La vie du Marquis de Sade. Paris, Gallimard, 1957

Lifton RJ: The Nazi Doctors. New York, Basic Books, 1986

Lloyd D: Ritual child abuse: understanding the controversies. Family Violence Bulletin, December 1990, pp 15–17

Lynch L: The Marquis de Sade. Boston, MA, Twayne, 1984

Masson J: The Assault on Truth. New York, Farrar, Straus & Giroux, 1984

Miller A: For Your Own Good: Hidden Cruelty in Child-Rearing and the Roots of Violence. New York, Farrar, Straus & Giroux, 1983

Nadelson T: Attachment to killing. Paper presented at the annual meeting of the American Academy of Psychoanalysis, New Orleans, LA, May 1–3, 1991

Ravenscroft T: The Spear of Destiny. New York, Putnam, 1973

Sartre JP: Saint Genet: Actor and Martyr. New York, Braziller, 1963

Schreiber F: Sybil. Chicago, IL, Regnery, 1973

Schreiber F, Arieti S: Multiple murders of a schizophrenic patient: a psychodynamic interpretation. J Am Acad Psychoanal 9:501–524, 1981

Smith SM, Hanson R, Noble S: Parents of battered babies: a controlled study. BMJ 4:388–391, 1974

Snow B, Sorensen T: Ritualistic child abuse in a neighborhood setting. Journal of Interpersonal Violence 5:474–487, 1990

Spengler A: Manifest sadomasochism of males: results of an empirical study. Arch Sex Behav 6:441–456, 1977

Stover E, Nightingale EO: The Breaking of Bodies and Minds. New York, Freeman, 1985

Suedfeld P: Psychology and Torture. New York, Hemisphere, 1990

Terry M: The Ultimate Evil: An Investigation of America's Most Dangerous Satanic Cult. Garden City, NY, Doubleday, 1987

van Benschoten SC: Multiple personality disorder and satanic ritual abuse: the issue of credibility. Dissociation 3:22–28, 1990

Wood WA, Hatton L: Triumph Over Darkness. Hillsboro, OR, Beyond Words, 1989

Young W, Sachs RG, Braun B, et al: Patients reporting ritual abuse in childhood: a clinical syndrome; report of 37 cases. Child Abuse Negl 15:181–189, 1991

Section IV

Grand Hysteria, Multiple Personality, and the Discovery of the Unconscious

> The same thing is happening to me as happens to people in dreams when they see and feel a wound but can't remember having received it.
>
> Alexander Dumas, *The Count of Monte Cristo*

> Visualizing mental formations, either voluntarily or not, is a most mysterious process. What becomes of these creatures? May it not be that like children born of our flesh, these children of our mind separate their lives from ours, escape our control and play parts of their own?
>
> Alexandra David-Neel
> *Magic and Mystery in Ancient Tibet*

Editor's Introduction

Ellenberger (1970) has described elegantly the intellectual excitement that grew in the nineteenth century as new case descriptions expanded understanding of the effects of the unconscious mind on body symptoms and on changes in self-states, manifested in behavior, emotion, and identity. The two early cases discussed here take us to the very beginning of this era, at the close of the eighteenth century.

It is 1791. The Marquis de Sade is temporarily at liberty in Paris, a revolutionary celebrity about to embark on his brief career as a judge. In Vienna, Mozart is dying. In America, the Bill of Rights becomes law. In Birmingham, England, Mary Reynolds is a child of 5. Her progressive Protestant relatives and their friends are in the midst of celebrating the second anniversary of the storming of the Bastille when an ugly riot begins to mobilize against them. This riot ushers in years of persecution and exile for Mary and her family, in the process of which Mary will develop the dissociative symptoms that are to carve her place in history. In 1791, yet another player in this epic is active. Anton Mesmer is wandering Europe under an assumed name, fleeing charges that his hypnotic treatment is quackery and rumors that he has sexually exploited patients. Doctor Guillotin had served on the Paris commission that condemned Mesmer (as had Benjamin Franklin and Lavoisier). By 1791, Mesmer might have been able to gain some ironic satisfaction from contemplating the ill effects of his accuser's invention, the guillotine, in comparison with the less tangible side effects of mesmerism. Both Estelle and, more tangentially, Mary Reynolds had connections with followers of Mesmer who were able to approach their somatic symptoms and their self-state changes in helpful ways, because similar phenomena had been observed under hypnosis.

Mary's tangential connection with Mesmer came through the Lunar Society, a group of Birmingham intellectuals who met each month on the Monday following the full moon to discuss new ideas in science, philosophy, and applied technology. The group included Josiah Wedgewood, owner of the Wedgewood Pottery; Joseph Priestley, the discoverer of oxygen; William Withering, discoverer of digitalis; and James Watt, inventor of the steam engine, as well as less well-known and occasional members like Mary Reynolds' uncle, who was a bookseller and historian. These intellectuals were specifically targeted in the Birmingham Riots, and many emigrated after rioters destroyed their homes and laboratories and their sense of intellectual and religious freedom (Goodwin 1987).

Erasmus Darwin, uncle of Charles Darwin and dabbler in mesmerism, was one of the members of the Lunar Society. In 1801, he published a study of one of the first cases of multiple personality disorder. As always in these early cases, there is a frustrating lack of childhood history so we do not know if this patient "with two minds" (like Mary Reynolds, who fell ill 10 years after Darwin's case was published) had also been a victim of the Birmingham Riots (Ellenberger 1970). Mary herself, living far away in the American wilderness, escaped hypnosis, and her successful diagnosis and treatment without that modality is one aspect of her case that continues to teach us.

By the end of the 19th century, some believed that this syndrome of perplexing multiple somatic symptoms and state changes at last had been catalogued and understood. At the Salpêtrière, Charcot could induce at will in his patients hysterical paralysis or the florid somatic symptoms of grand hysteria. He could also lead his patients through the various states of consciousness that characterized his version of hypnosis. However, after Charcot's death, these certainties dissolved. It was found that Salpêtrière patients could be induced to perform grand hysteria for the price of a few coins, and staff members admitted having tutored them to pantomime correctly the various hypnotic stages.

What would have served as an anchor here was trauma, that quantity that Charcot and his predecessors so persistently left out of their formulations. Always in these patients, muttered Charcot to his student Freud, there is the sexual thing. If he knows that, thought Freud, why doesn't he ever talk about it? In truth, when one reads the case studies from the Salpêtrière, one finds the sexual thing routinely—and one finds, as well, the neglect thing, the battering thing, the parental addiction or psychosis thing, and the sadism thing. Consider the patient Louise, whose hysterical paralysis, anesthesia, and seizures were the subjects of Charcot's phenomenologic interest. Charcot's lectures covered those points extensively, but not the circumstances of her life: that five of her six siblings died in childhood, that she had been punished by being locked in a room, that her mother's boyfriend raped her, and that she had made her living as a prostitute since age 13 (Goodwin 1989).

Without the concrete details of the childhood trauma to anchor us, all we have is a patient whose physical and psychic pain are extreme and who is seriously confused about every aspect of that pain because of amnesia and other dissociative symptoms. We have a pain preparation in search of a diagnosis. Under such circumstances, we make errors in diagnosis. "Grand hysteria" is as much a misdiagnosis as the neurological diagnoses that were made in the cases of Mary Reynolds and Estelle. Today's stock diagnoses—"borderline" or "schizoaffective"—are in many cases equally wrong. Such patients may seek explanations for their pain in "past-life trauma," tales of contact with flying saucers or in the pseudoexplanation of demon possession (see Chapters 3 and 4). The patient is grateful for any diagnosis that allows him or her to bypass the treacherous territory of childhood experience of pain, betrayal, and abandonment.

What is even more remarkable, though, is how responsive to treatment these patients remain even when their physicians are entirely off the track. Louise improved in the Salpêtrière, and Mary Reynolds and Estelle achieved excellent symptom control despite (or perhaps because of) the diagnostic and therapeutic naivete of their physicians (although Despine had seen similar cases). The therapeutic lessons in these cases remind us to cleave to the basics with such patients: Respect the patient's requests and personal metaphors about cure, attend to the somatic symptoms and follow them up with complete physical examination, and insist on filling in the amnestic gaps in the patient's life history. The latter will often require the collection of documents, records, and interviews both from the patient's family and other collateral informants. What we often learn once we collect these concrete data is how far the patient has drifted from the realities of his or her own lived pain and how necessary our misdiagnoses have become in helping to maintain that distance (Goodwin 1988).

References

Ellenberger H: The Discovery of the Unconscious: The History and Evolution of Dynamic Psychiatry. New York, Basic Books, 1970

Goodwin J: Mary Reynolds: a post-traumatic reinterpretation of a classic case of multiple personality disorder. Hillside J Clin Psychiatry 9:89–99, 1987

Goodwin J: Munchausen's syndrome as a dissociative sequel to extreme child abuse. Dissociation 1:54–60, 1988

Goodwin J: Sexual Abuse: Incest Victims and Their Families. Chicago, IL, Mosby Yearbook, 1989

Chapter 6

Mary Reynolds and Estelle: Somatic Symptoms and Unacknowledged Trauma

Jean M. Goodwin, M.D., M.P.H.
Catherine Fine, Ph.D.

Despite the widespread impression that multiple personality disorder is a new and thereby suspect diagnosis, the first cases were described in the medical literature in the early nineteenth century.

The first American case was Mary Reynolds, a young woman on the American frontier who fell ill in 1811. The first child case was 10-year-old Estelle, who fell ill in 1834 and was treated at a French health spa. Both cases featured numerous and florid physical symptoms. Mary Reynolds became blind and deaf for several months. Estelle had been paralyzed for 2 years when she sought treatment and suffered numerous other somatic symptoms. Neurological diagnoses were considered in both cases.

In both early cases, there was a history of severe trauma; however, this was never brought into focus by the patients' physicians or connected to their symptoms. Mary Reynolds went through two sets of religious riots in her home in Birmingham, England, before her family fled to America when she was 8. Despite this, her medical biographer Weir Mitchell (1888) pronounced her childhood to have been "marked by no extraordinary incidents" (p. 368). In fact, the traumatic nature of the family's plight as a persecuted religious minority and as refugees has been revealed only through much more recent research into family memoirs and documents (Carlson 1984; Goodwin 1987). Estelle's exposure to medical trauma included her own bout of measles encephalitis at age 5 and her witnessing at age 7 a cholera epidemic that killed her father and almost killed her mother and sister (Despine 1840; Fine 1988).

Associated findings in both cases are familiar to present-day clinicians and include amnesia, ego fragmentation and splitting, depression and self-destructive behavior, anxiety symptoms, and a proneness to argument and relapse that led both patients to be labelled as difficult. Despite these multiple problems, both patients were treated by general practitioners who achieved significant steps toward cure for both.

In this chapter, we describe each historical case and discuss the numerous somatic symptoms and the unacknowledged trauma found in each case as clues of continuing importance in the diagnoses of severe posttraumatic syndromes complicated by amnesia and other forms of dissociation. Such individuals have amnesia and confusion not only for their personal history but also for their present symptoms. This makes them vulnerable to misdiagnosis unless the clinician pursues a thorough evaluation, including physical examination; laboratory testing; interview of collateral informants; and collection of medical records and other relevant documents, such as birth and death certificates, school records, and family photographs and memorabilia.

The Case of Mary Reynolds

Mary Reynolds was a chronically depressed 25-year-old single woman living on a Pennsylvania frontier farm with her parents. The family had arrived at the farm 12 years previously, in 1798, after a 4-year exodus from their home in Birmingham, England. In Birmingham, their home had been looted and their church had been burned, with similar damage done to homes and businesses belonging to friends and relatives, in two major riots in 1791 and 1793. The riots were aimed at the non-Anglican "dissenting" Protestant minority; both Mary's father and grandfather were dissenting ministers. Her father was also a friend of Joseph Priestley, the main target of the riots. Eight younger siblings had been born during Mary's first 16 chaotic years; one died between the first and second riots. Mary had become more withdrawn and hyperreligious after her older sister's death from smallpox in 1804. She also worried about rumors of war between her adopted and native countries (Kenny 1986); the rumored hostilities were soon to erupt into the War of 1812.

In 1810, Mary was found lying in the fields unconscious, in an apparent seizure. She remained blind and deaf for 6 weeks before returning to her usual state. Her somnolence and loss of perception somewhat resembled an epidemic of religious cataplexy that had passed through the neighborhood some years before (Reynolds 1938) except that Mary's episode was much more prolonged.

Three months later, Mary was again found in a seizurelike sleep. This time she woke as an infant who had to be retaught to eat, to say the names of family members, to speak, and finally to recite the alphabet (Goodrich-Freer 1907).

Over the next 13 years, Mary shifted back and forth every 5 or 6 weeks between her original state (State A) and this second, "younger" Mary (State B). In State A, she had phobias and anxiety as well as melancholy, sometimes trembling so violently that her bed would shake. She was sickly and had excruciating headaches; at times, she was bedridden for weeks. She was described as sober and "a slow thinker devoid of imagination" (Plumer 1860, p. 808). State A had no memories of State B and lived in despair and dread of switching; State B had no memories of State A. However, Mary in State B was blissfully unafraid even of such realistic hazards as bears, crossing thin ice, and rattlesnakes (she followed one to its hole and reached in with her hand to catch the pretty thing). Her physician had great difficulty keeping the "younger" Mary out of physical danger. Mary B mocked Mary A's preoccupation with loss and the whole family's melancholy tone. She referred to the family home as "The Nocturnal Shades." Mary B loved company and practical jokes and was a good poet. Her physician was often the butt of her wit. She often forgot to eat or sleep. Eventually Mary stabilized in a third state best described as a more adult Mary B. She wrote about her initial exuberance: "Had all my friends been lying dead beside me, I do not think I would have experienced one moment's pain" (Mitchell 1888, p. 378).

Although the "younger" Mary had no memories of Birmingham, she had dreams of places that family members were able to recognize (as their now destroyed church) and of people that Mary had known in England. In a series of recurrent dreams, Mary's dead sister Eliza came to reeducate Mary in Christianity. "I love to dream of her," wrote Mary B in her diary, "though when awake I have not the slightest recollection of her" (Plumer 1860, p. 810).

In the process of settling into the Mary B identity, Mary neatly excised 8 years from her age and life history. Those who knew Mary in later life listed her birthdate as 1793 (Plumer 1860). However, birth records in England list her date of birth as September 18, 1785 (Carlson

1984; Goodrich-Freer 1907). Mary compounded the confusion about her birthdate by telling suitors she was "360."

What Mary achieved in her illness was the extirpation of the Birmingham years and the riots from her life. Also apparently excised were feelings of fear, loss, and anger connected with the family's experience of discrimination and religious persecution. Sketches of her by contemporaries are not detailed enough to tell us whether Mary B had substituted an American accent for Mary A's old Birmingham one in the process of relearning language. We know that the A and B handwritings differed significantly and that family members recognized the personality shift instantaneously. Also, we are told that Mary B had no fear of the American wilderness that the actual 12-year-old child Mary had entered with her mother in such loneliness and dread. This is her brother's description of that moment: "When the child asked, 'Mother, is this home?' she (mother) replied by a gush of tears, unable otherwise to answer. All the sweet memories of friends far distant, of church associations, of the thousand nameless comforts of former home ties, would . . . make the present moment inexpressibly painful" (Reynolds 1938, p. 79). Mary's illness had put all of this far behind her. The 4-year splitting up of family members (brother and father had gone on ahead), the painful move, the month's voyage by boat and cart through uncharted areas infested by wolves and hostile Indians—all this was displaced into Mary's infancy rather than experienced as disrupting her latency years, when homesickness and nostalgia for childhood are factors even under the most favorable external circumstances. What is also remarkable is that those around Mary cooperated with this extirpation so completely that no mention of the riots or the trauma of the relocation appears in her medical history.

Several circumstances in addition to her own extirpation of her traumatic history may have facilitated Mary's recovery. Her illness propelled her out of her home, first to live with a brother and sister-in-law (who was the widow of Mary's first physician). However, she began to thrive when she began work as her nephew's housekeeper; he was a minister and one of the founders of Allegheny College in Pennsylvania. Mary Reynolds seems to have settled down within the structure of college life, surrounded by young people—perhaps in a similar way to Christoph Haizmann (see Chapter 3), who found peace in monastic life. In this process, too, Mary Reynolds was able to contribute in her own small way to reconstructing in a safer place the spirit of open inquiry and free exploration that had been destroyed in the Birmingham Riots.

The Case of Estelle

In the summer of 1836, 11-year-old Estelle was brought from Switzerland to a French health spa for treatment of paralysis, which she had had for 2 years and which had been diagnosed as a spinal cord lesion; she also experienced skin neuralgia, which made every touch excruciating. In addition, she had a painful inability to warm herself, bizarre eating habits (she could tolerate only a few foods), frequent headaches, nervous cough, pressure on her chest, and abdominal pain. Estelle had been around illness much of her life. At age 5 she almost died of measles encephalitis; at age 7, she had watched her family succumb to cholera, which killed her father. Estelle made the trip to the spa by train lying in a darkened coach in a large willow basket padded with eiderdown. If anyone other than her mother or aunt touched her, she would scream. Estelle's mental status included, in addition to her spoiled demandingness, absorption in daydreams, hallucinations, thoughts of death, and amnesia so extreme that she could not reconstruct her daily activities.

Despine (1840) was the general physician in charge of the thermal station to which Estelle was brought. He instituted a program of hydrotherapy and electrical treatment. After several months, he learned from Estelle's mother that Estelle conversed at night with a choir of angels. The mother thought these were the angelic companions of Estelle's dead father. Despine resolved to use magnetism to explore this. Estelle agreed only if she could have control of the timing and depth of trance and only if everything she said in trance would be repeated to her word for word. The mother took charge of keeping a treatment diary that facilitated this latter request.

Using trance, Despine was able to contact four angels and several other companions of Estelle's, including a skeleton, an old dead woman, fighting couples, and men who made scary grimaces. One of the angels, Angeline, conversed with Estelle and Despine and was even more insistent than Estelle had been about dictating conditions for treatment. These suggestions included—again, rather sensibly—not forcing Estelle to eat foods that she did not like. Within a month, the Angeline-Estelle state had developed its own behaviors as well as opinions. In this state, Estelle could walk, run, travel tirelessly, play, and eat everything. For the first time in her life, she displayed anger openly. In her normal state, Estelle remained a bedridden invalid, morbidly dependent on her mother. The Angeline state could not tolerate the mother and much preferred Despine.

By the fourth month of treatment, Angeline-Estelle orchestrated her own integration, visualizing a big ball that was to burst inside her, breaking through walls of amnesia (Ellenberger 1970; Fine 1988). At this point, somatic symptoms resolved in all states.

After a year's treatment at the thermal baths, which had included 6 months of hypnotic treatment, Estelle returned home to Switzerland symptom-free, except that her fear of cats remained and occasionally triggered a cataleptic trance. She later married, and she died at age 37.

Somatic Symptoms as Clues to Childhood Trauma

Mary Reynolds's recorded somatic symptoms include pseudoseizures, hysterical blindness, hysterical deafness, headache, catatonia, inability to speak, inability to write, shivering, and general sickliness. Estelle had hysterical paralysis, chronic pain, shivering, headaches, abdominal pain, chest pressure, and nervous cough. Both had odd eating habits, with Mary B forgetting to eat and with Estelle refusing almost all foods. Both were seriously disabled by amnesia.

The multiplicity of somatic symptoms and the recurrence of certain specific complaints in both cases recall somatic syndromes discussed in previous chapters in this book. Electra complained of headache, easy startle, and emaciation. The seventeenth-century painter Christoph Haizmann had pseudoseizures, sensory disturbances, and shivering. In these very early cases, the reporters' delicacy usually precludes listing genital, anal, or menstrual symptoms. A similar litany of somatic symptoms will be found both in Anna O and Dora (Chapters 7 and 8) and in the case from *I Never Promised You a Rose Garden* described in Chapter 9.

Today, the presence of multiple symptoms in a setting of anxiety, depression, and disturbed relationships and self-concept would prompt us to screen for Briquet's Syndrome or Somatization Disorder. Criteria for this disorder involve both the presence of a multiplicity of symptoms and the presence of certain core symptoms found with highest frequency. These core symptoms include pain in the extremities, shortness of breath, difficulty swallowing, vomiting, genital or anal burning, menstrual pain, and amnesia. It is remarkable that these seven symptoms, selected statistically on the basis of high frequency in recent American samples, are precisely the symptoms one would expect in a sexual abuse victim (Goodwin, in press). In sexual abuse, the victim's arms and legs are held down. The body weight of the assailant presses down on the victim's chest and interferes with breathing. Oral penetration leads to difficulty swallowing; ejaculation into the mouth may produce gagging and vomiting; anal or vaginal penetration may lead to burning and at times to deep pain, which is often experienced around menses. All or part of the experience may be blotted out by amnesia, especially if there is the threat of death if the victim discloses.

A trauma theorist (Loewenstein 1990) is not surprised to learn that more than half of these somatizing patients describe sexual molestation in childhood (Morrison 1989) nor to learn that similar symptoms are described acutely by rape victims (Weigandt et al. 1990). Somatic symptoms have long been understood as markers for sexual traumata. Freud listed genital paresthesias, urinary symptoms, intestinal symptoms, choking, vomiting, and food refusal as symptoms found in his series of 18 adult victims of childhood sexual abuse (Freud 1896/1958). Briquet's original (1859) publication describes a history of family violence in 27% of patients with multiple somatic symptoms. The very term "hysteria" derives from the name of a sexual orgy held in honor of Aphrodite at the New Year. Physicians named the syndrome of sequelae after the orgy these patients had attended (Macalpine and Hunter 1960).

For Mary Reynolds and Estelle, we need not postulate occult sexual abuse to understand their somatic symptoms (although because this history was not explicitly screened for, it could well have been present in both). Known trauma in both cases illuminates the symptoms.

In Mary's case, we know that rioters looted Mary's own home and threatened to burn it (Goodrich-Freer 1907). We also have a graphic account of the experience of the riots from Mary's aunt (Hutton 1875). Catherine Hutton describes hearing about the riots, seeing flames, fleeing, and being turned out of several inns where her family sought shelter. She and her family were hiding in another inn when a party of rioters entered:

> They entered the house, and I heard them swear they believed some Presbyterian was inside, and they would either burn it or pull it down. I expected every moment that we would be betrayed. . . . For two hours we remained speechless and immovable. (Hutton 1875, p. 20)

Years later, in Mary we see inability to speak and seizures that leave her immobilized except for shivering as if in great fear. One could speculate that her blindness and deafness reflected efforts to "turn off" frightening auditory and visual flashbacks.

Estelle had experienced measles encephalitis, with the death threat of the disease reinforced by witnessing the cholera death of her father. Subsequently, she experienced headaches, an inability to move, shivering, and failure to thermoregulate. (Chapter 9 describes symptoms in another victim whose primary childhood trauma was medical illness.) In addition to reexperiencing the somatic symptoms of illness, Estelle reenacted the trauma of treatment, dreading both inflicted pain by her caretakers and overcontrol.

The Importance of Medical and Pediatric Records and the Physical Examination

Assembly of all medical records should be routine when multiple somatic symptoms and amnesia coincide. Despine (1840) was fortunate to have access to Estelle's mother, who provided the personal and familial medical history. The pediatric history can provide indicators to neglect such as absent immunizations, recurrent pneumonia, or failure to thrive. Notes in school or pediatric records can also document early symptoms secondary to childhood abuse. One patient had sustained recurrent hospitalizations for getting his hand "caught" in the washer-wringer and still another hospitalization for swollen and bruised genitals secondary to a beating. The therapist often finds recurrent pediatric visits for vaginal discharge or urinary tract infection in patients later recovering memories of sexual abuse.

In cases of sadistic abuse, the physical examination may yield clarifying data, including scars, evidence of prior vaginal intercourse or pregnancy for which the victim is amnestic, or excision of genital landmarks such as nipples, clitoris, or labia. In one patient who had described being disciplined by having pins stuck under her skin, we found one of the pins on radiographic survey.

How Childhood Trauma Vanishes

Many victims face specific prohibitions against speaking about or even knowing about childhood trauma. The shame and guilt that surround parental physical or sexual abuse are well known. Under these circumstances, multiple environmental cues encourage the child to forget the victimization. In some families, a particular lie may be sustained for years to conceal, for example, an adoption or an illegitimate pregnancy or a family member's mental illness, alcoholism, imprisonment, or suicide. The very fact of victimization is shameful in our society, especially for men, and victims tend to be blamed. Even when the abuser is a nonfamily member, shame and silence may condition the family's response, especially if the family is involved in some secret, clandestine, or criminal activity or if family members feel guilt on some irrational basis.

For Mary Reynolds and Estelle, it is not clear how shame and secrecy operated to help their traumata disappear. What is clear in both these cases is that space and time were working against these young women and had become obstacles to the grieving process.

Both had moved away from the site of the trauma—Mary from England to America and Estelle from Switzerland to France. Such drastic moves facilitate distancing from the trauma and numbing, removing the victim from the sensory triggers that can revivify fragmented memories and provide opportunities for reintegration. It may have helped Estelle to be brought back to France for treatment. In addition, both victims were more than 2 years distant in time from the overwhelming event, and both had lost important potential confidantes—Mary her sister and Estelle her father. In the first 2 years after a family tragedy, it is relatively easy to bring up the loss. For example, in the first years after the Reynolds family moved, they entertained many visitors from Birmingham, including Wedgewood's son. However, 12 years later, 5 years later, the interests of other family members have moved on. In their illnesses, Mary and Estelle had to invent confidantes who would have the requisite knowledge and interest to share their grief. Mary spoke to her dead sister in dreams, and Estelle gained access to her father through the angel Angeline.

In neither of these historical cases was the childhood trauma reconstructed in psychotherapy. However, in both cases the trauma was reenacted in the (not yet named or discovered) "transference." Mary

Reynolds repeatedly tested her physician to see if he could keep her safe from wandering off and getting lost or hurt in a hostile environment. Estelle tested Despine as to whether he could be a good doctor who would explain what was happening, allow her some physical freedom, and meet her basic needs without increasing her pain. One can imagine that Mary's physician was dealing at times with a 5-year-old terrorized by a riot and that Despine at times was talking with a 5-year-old terrorized by a near-fatal illness. In both cases, there was immersion in a therapeutic milieu, with Estelle living at the spa and with Mary's entire community conspiring in her treatment.

The Importance of Documents and Collateral Informants

Rosenzweig (1987) uses the term "psychoarcheology" to describe the painstaking research required to reconstruct family and life histories in these famous historical cases. One locates birth and death certificates, memoirs, school and medical records, letters, local histories, police records, and contemporary newspapers. Rosenzweig studied the case of "Sally Beauchamp," whose multiple personality disorder was treated by Morton Prince, a Boston neurologist, at the turn of the century. Using psychoarcheology, Rosenzweig discovered traumata that Prince had never uncovered. "Sally," at age 7, had an infant sister who died. A similar infant death followed by the mother's death took place later when "Sally" was 13, and this later trauma did become a focus of Prince's treatment. The earlier death that Prince never uncovered probably intensified the impact of the second loss (see Chapter 4). Rosenzweig also discovered that "Sally" had extensive school absences after her mother's death and that at age 15, "Sally" ran away from home and never recontacted her father during the last 30 years of his life. These circumstances raise the question of whether "Sally" had to replace her mother in a domestic sense and perhaps in a sexual sense, which she countered by running away and severing contact.

The psychoarcheological approach is just as necessary in clinical cases as it is in these historical ones. In one case, a careful family history revealed five suicides among first- and second-degree relatives. Another patient brought in a family photograph that depicted four generations of women in her family, intoxicated and drinking alcohol;

the patient was 5 years old at the time of the photograph. Memorabilia are often helpful in reconstruction. One patient had saved a lock of her hair from childhood. As she reconstructed her father's perversion, which involved his ejaculating into her hair, we submitted the keepsake to chemical analysis, which revealed the presence of semen. Another patient with fragmented memories of bizarre sex acts had saved a matchbox; the hotel named on the matchbox was a known site for the filming of pornography.

Forensic psychiatry and child guidance have always emphasized the use of collateral informants and documents. In patients with amnesia, such sources are indispensable.

Conclusion

The copresence of multiple somatic symptoms and inability to describe one's own emotional life was described in the mid-twentieth century as alexithymia (Sifneos 1973). Similarly frustrating clinical pictures have been described in Holocaust victims (Bergmann and Jucovy 1982). The two patients whose cases were described in this chapter were cut off by amnesia and family circumstances from their personal history as well as their emotions. Their illnesses allowed them to regress to the developmental state at which the initial trauma occurred and to reexperience the somatic and emotional pain they had suffered. They created imaginary companions who had the knowledge to act as confidantes. Fears and wishes related to the initial trauma were enacted in their relationships with their physicians.

Mary Reynolds, whose adult life is better known, can be seen as devoting her life after recovery to reconstructing what had been destroyed in the traumatic Birmingham riots. Her story provides an object lesson in the difficulty of defining one of these patients as "nonabused." Mary was so defined, and by Weir Mitchell (who was a most careful clinician), despite the fact that the Birmingham Riots constituted a trauma so public that they can still be reconstructed through documents 200 years later.

References

Bergmann S, Jucovy ME: Generations of the Holocaust. New York, Basic Books, 1982

Briquet P: Traité de l'Hystérie. Paris, Bailliere, 1859

Carlson T: The history of multiple personality in the United States: Mary Reynolds and her subsequent reputation. Bull Hist Med 58:72–82, 1984

Despine A: De l'emploi de magnétisme animal et des eaux minérales dans le traitment des maladies nerveuses, suivie d'une observation très curieuse de neuropathie. Paris, Baillière, 1840

Ellenberger H: The Discovery of the Unconscious: The History and Evolution of Dynamic Psychiatry. New York, Basic Books, 1970

Fine C: The work of Antoine Despine: the first scientific report on the diagnosis and treatment of a child with multiple personality disorder. Am J Clin Hypn 31:33–39, 1988

Freud S: The aetiology of hysteria (1896), in the Standard Edition of the Complete Psychological Works of Sigmund Freud, Vol 3. Translated and edited by J Strachey. London, Hogarth Press, 1958, pp 187–221

Goodrich-Freer AM: A case of double personality. Occult Review 5:95–104, 1907

Goodwin J: Mary Reynolds: a post-traumatic reinterpretation of a classic case of multiple personality disorder. Hillside J Clin Psychiatry 9:89–99, 1987

Goodwin J: Childhood sexual abuse in psychogenic non-epileptic seizures, in The Dilemma of Non-Epileptic Seizures. Edited by Rowan AJ. New York, Butterworth Heineman (in press)

Hutton C: A Narrative of the Riots in Birmingham, July, 1791. Birmingham, England, White & Pike, 1875

Kenny MG: The Passion of Ansel Bourne: Multiple Personality in American Culture. Washington, DC, Smithsonian, 1986

Loewenstein R: Somatoform disorders in victims of incest and child abuse, in Incest-Related Syndromes of Adult Psychopathology. Edited by Kluft RP. Washington DC, American Psychiatric Press, 1990, pp 75–112

Macalpine I, Hunter RA: Schizophrenia 1677. London, Dawson, 1960

Mitchell SW: Mary Reynolds: a case of double consciousness. Transactions of the College of Physicians of Philadelphia 10:366–389, 1888

Morrison J: Childhood sexual histories in women with somatization disorder. Am J Psychiatry 146:239–241, 1989

Plumer S: Mary Reynolds: a case of double consciousness. Harper's New Monthly Magazine 20:807–812, 1860

Reynolds JE: In French Creek Valley. Meadville, PA, Crawford County Historical Society, 1938

Rosenzweig S: Sally Beauchamp's career: a psychoarcheological key to Morton Prince's classic case of multiple personality. Genet Soc Gen Psychol Monogr 113:5–60, 1987

Sifneos P: The prevalence of alexithymic characteristics in psychosomatic patients, in Psychotherapy in Psychosomatics. Edited by Reusch J, Schmale A, Spoerri T. White Plains, NY, Karger, 1973, pp 255–262

Weigandt A, Wallace DL, Phelps L, et al: The impact of sexual assault on physical health status. Journal of Traumatic Stress 3:93–102, 1990

Section V

Early Psychoanalytic Cases

> Every man's life is a solution in hieroglyphic to those inquiries he would put. He acts it in life before he apprehends it as truth.
>
> Emerson, *The Conduct of Life*

> He wasn't clever at all: he merely told
> The unhappy Present to recite the Past
> Like a poetry lesson till sooner
> Or later it faltered at the line where,
> Long ago, the accusations had begun. . . .
>
> W. H. Auden on Freud, *Collected Poems*

Editor's Introduction

In the 1980s, controversy about Jeffrey Masson's book *The Assault on Truth* (1984) seemed to cast Sigmund Freud as an adversary of trauma theory. Viewed in historical perspective, however, it becomes clear that Freud and Breuer, his mentor and collaborator, took revolutionary steps toward forging definitive connections between the mysterious symptoms in their patients and the patients' previously experienced traumata.

The two young women whose treatments are reviewed in this section presented with symptoms similar to those described in Chapter 6. Both Anna O and Dora complained of difficulty breathing, nervous cough, loss of voice, seizurelike episodes, headache, and facial pain. In addition, each had her own unique list of additional somatic symptoms. Both were survivors of documented sociopolitical and medical traumata. As Jews, both underwent constant social and political discrimination, which Breuer and Freud, as its covictims, may have minimized. Anna O would become a crusader against the political, economic, and sexual exploitation of Jewish women; later, Dora, despite having converted to Christianity, would barely escape the Holocaust, losing almost everything except her life (Decker 1991). Anna O nursed her father through his last illness. Dora, at an even earlier age, nursed her father when he was ill with syphilis, then tuberculosis, and then a detached retina. Dora's own illnesses had led to drastic interventions, including electrotherapy and cold water treatments, as she was growing up in the hospital-like environment of a health resort for people with tuberculosis.

In both cases, present-day reviewers have asked whether these young women experienced child abuse beyond the known extrafamilial and medical traumata. One does not need to extrapolate far from the data to ask whether these two women were being emotionally abused and exploited to fulfill their parents' aims while their own developmental needs were neglected and ignored. It must have been painful both for Dora and Anna O to compare their own opportunities with those of their brothers, who had access to wider options along any dimension: education, travel, social connections, work, and political expression.

We can only speculate about the presence of overt sexual abuse in these cases. We know that present-day victims of childhood sexual abuse have symptoms quite similar to those found in Anna O and Dora: suicidality, depression, nightmares, intrusive memories, disordered eating, and multiple somatic symptoms, especially pseudoseizures (Goodwin 1990). Anna O's later pseudopregnancy and her interest in "white slavery" and Dora's lifelong unexplained vaginal discharge are the kinds of specific sexual sublimations and symptoms that sometimes recur in victims of overt or covert incest. However, there is no magic in a sexual abuse history. Sexual abuse is often found in association with severe symptoms, because it is such a severe and multiple trauma source, providing in one package physical abuse, emotional neglect, sexual overstimulation, blaming, exploitation, isolation, death threat, and witnessing of parental emotional dyscontrol and spousal conflict. Similar traumatic input can come in other forms. I recall a child custody case in which the judge was interested only in whether the mother's allegations of paternal incest were provable. It was considered irrelevant that the father when angry would put a revolver to the mother's head and threaten to kill her and then the child.

There are differences in the two cases as well. Anna O had more problems with dissociation. Although both became at times dazed, depersonalized, and derealized, Anna O was amnestic for much of her day and entered split-off ego states in which she lost access to large sectors of her own feelings, body sensations, memories, or behaviors, as the ability to speak her own tongue.

There are also differences in treatment. Breuer was a general practitioner doing his best to respond helpfully to Anna O's severe psychiatric symptoms. This was also the tradition of Despine, who prescribed rest, baths, and mineral water. It was this eclectic clinical pragmatism that gave birth to the "talking cure." The discovery was not without its price, a price perhaps best described by Breuer himself:

> At that time I learned something of practical importance . . . namely, that it was impossible for a general practitioner to treat a case of that kind without bringing his activities and mode of life completely to an end. I vowed at the time I would *not* go through such an ordeal again. (Cranefeld 1958, p. 319)

It is important to appreciate Breuer's first attempt at psychotherapy in the same way we would other nineteenth-century medical breakthroughs: the first use of intravenous fluids or the first mastectomy for cancer. It goes without saying that the technique was crude. It can also be assumed that both physician and index patient were unique individuals involved in a relationship extraordinary enough to inspire an absolutely new solution. One factor that has been noted in the Breuer–Anna O relationship is that her real name, Bertha, was the same as Breuer's mother's name; Breuer's mother had died when he was 3 and when his mother had been the same age as Anna O was at the time she came for treatment (Dexter 1991).

Loewenstein's chapter on Anna O (Chapter 7) highlights the association between her father's terminal illness and the emergence of her severe symptoms. He notes that this is a pattern often seen in abuse victims. Indeed, it is a pattern in evidence throughout this book. Oedipus's father dies; Electra's father dies; the seventeenth-century painter's father dies; Avraham's father dies; Estelle's father dies. Whether the parent figure is seen as an abuser, a protector, or a witness, the loss may precipitate profound disequilibrium and new symptoms.

In many ways, Dora can be understood as the daughter of Anna O. Some think Freud chose the fictitious name "Dora" in part because this young patient was born in the same year as his friend's child, Dora Breuer, the daughter conceived during that much-discussed interlude when Breuer withdrew from the intensity of treating Anna O and took a vacation with his wife (Decker 1991).

In our discussion of Dora, we focus on understanding her "resistances" not as noncompliance but as intelligible sequelae of her trauma. Of course, she experienced the treatment as a repetition of the sexual exploitation she had endured. Of course she tried to protect herself with every ounce of recalcitrance she could muster. Of course she cared more about repairing her parents than herself. Of course she experienced sexuality more as a child than an adult. Of course she lived in a state of chronic rage. Freud hoped she could let go of some of these behaviors so they could begin treatment; Dora tried to explain that doing this was the only way she knew to begin. I am reminded of a patient of mine, a chronic self-mutilator, who threw back her head and laughed when I asked her to sign a "No Harm Contract" (Braun 1986) so that we could begin treatment. "I won't be able to sign this until I'm well," she explained.

Both Breuer and Freud lost their patients to treatment, Breuer after a year and a half and Freud after only 3 months. Both physicians felt they had lost control of treatment and perhaps been wounded themselves in the process. Both were forced to confront their own obliviousness to the reenactments of sexual trauma in their treatment technique. Breuer was calling on his patient in her home, often in her bedroom, each evening. Freud instructed his patient to recline on his couch with her eyes closed while he talked explicitly with her about sexual matters.

Anna O was able to log more treatment hours than Dora and on lifetime follow-up may have done better than her spiritual daughter. The two women differed markedly in their response to anti-Semitism—Anna O becoming a champion of Jewish women, thereby founding social work, and Dora converting to Protestantism, probably in an attempt to spare her cherished son the discrimination she had endured. One recalls Dora describing to Freud the afternoon she had spent in rapt contemplation of a painting of the Madonna. Perhaps both of these patients were trying to reclaim and reconstruct the lost mothers who had failed to protect them. Anna O was perhaps luckier in being able to find not merely a symbol but flesh and blood female role models who helped her forge a network of relationships with other women (Herman 1992). Dora, too, had a relatively happy interlude in later life when she worked as a bridge mistress, playing cards each day in a mostly female milieu. Although Dora herself is renowned only as a patient, the men she loved best, her brother and her son, gained international respect for their work—one as a socialist politician and one as a classical conductor. Given such outcomes in the face of such overwhelming trauma and emotional pain, one hesitates to be too critical of these treatments, and one continues to ask what we can learn from them.

References

Braun B: Treatment of Multiple Personality Disorder. Washington, DC, American Psychiatric Association, 1986

Cranefeld P: Josef Breuer's evaluation of his contributions to psychoanalysis. Int J Psychoanal 39:319–322, 1958

Decker H: Freud, Dora, and Vienna 1900. New York, Free Press, 1991

Goodwin J: Borderline and other severe symptoms in adult survivors of sexual abuse. Psychiatric Annals 20:22–32, 1990

Herman JL: Trauma and Recovery. New York, Basic Books, 1992

Masson J: The Assault on Truth. New York, Farrar, Straus & Giroux, 1984

Chapter 7

Anna O: Reformulation as a Case of Multiple Personality Disorder

Richard J. Loewenstein, M.D.

> It is not, indeed, that I have never had to do with symptoms which demonstrably arose during dissociated states of consciousness and were obliged for that reason to remain excluded from the ego. . . . I was able to show afterwards that the so-called hypnoid state owed its separation to the fact that in it a psychical group had come into effect which had previously been split off by defense. In short, I am unable to suppress a suspicion that somewhere or other roots of hypnoid and defense hysteria come together, and that the primary factor is defense. (Freud, *Studies in Hysteria* [1895/1955a], p. 286)

The case of Anna O (Breuer and Freud 1893–1895/1955) is one of the most famous in the history of psychiatry and psychoanalysis. Over the years, it has fascinated clinicians to such an extent that numerous reinterpretations have been published. Anna O has received multiple diagnoses in the literature, including hysteria and hysterical psychosis (Freud 1910/1955b), "double personality" (Jones 1953), multiple personality (Ellenberger 1972; Kluft 1987; Nakdimen 1988), schizophrenia (Goshen 1952; Reichard 1956), melancholia and pathological mourning (Pollock 1972, 1984), hysterical personality (Bolkosky 1982), borderline disorder or borderline psychotic state (Gargiulo 1984; Meissner 1979; Spotnitz 1984), major depression, anxiety disorder, and conversion disorder (Martorano 1984), drug-induced delirium and complex partial seizures (Orr-Andrawes 1987), and spontaneous acute disseminated encephalomyelitis (Hurst 1982), among others.

In addition, the case has been reformulated according to family systems theory (Bloch 1984), discussed in terms of the cultural and intellectual history of late nineteenth-century Vienna (Bolkosky 1982; Ellenberger 1970, 1972; Macmillan 1977; Muroff 1984; Spiegel 1984), and reexamined from a feminist/historical perspective (Kaplan 1984; Steinmann 1984). There is even a study that compares the personality profile of Bertha Pappenheim—the woman who is thought to have been the actual Anna O—to that of contemporary American female social workers (Armbruster 1982). In addition, since Jones's (1953) disclosure of Anna O's apparent actual identity, much scholarship has been devoted to uncovering details of the life of Bertha Pappenheim (Edinger 1968; Ellenberger 1970, 1972; Freeman 1972; Hirschmuller 1989; Jensen 1970; Pollock 1968, 1972, 1984; Rosenbaum 1984).

This chapter has several purposes. First, I will take a phenomenological approach to the case, showing that the symptoms displayed by Anna O are most consistent with a diagnosis of a dissociative disorder, most probably multiple personality disorder (MPD). In addition, I will review the classical Anna O/Bertha Pappenheim (Anna O/Bertha P) "story" and some of the subsequent biographical scholarship on Anna O, Bertha Pappenheim, and Breuer to show that much of the psychodynamic data supports a diagnosis of MPD as well. I will give case examples from contemporary MPD patients to illustrate these points.

Retrospective reanalysis of historic psychiatric cases or of the lives of famous figures from the past (paleodiagnosis) has notable limitations—so much of the data is missing that would ordinarily be available in a contemporary clinical case. Often these retrospective case reports become like projective tests that say more about the contemporary reinterpreter than about the original participants in the case. The multiple reexaminations of the Anna O/Bertha P case often read like works of literary criticism in which a classical piece is repeatedly reinterpreted according to the dominant academic preoccupations of subsequent eras (see in particular Rosenbaum and Muroff 1984).

Despite these limitations, it is my hope that the current chapter will be persuasive in its diagnostic and dynamic formulations. In addition, I hope that my discussion may serve to illustrate some issues in clinical work with contemporary patients with MPD.

The Case of Anna O as Presented by Breuer and Freud

It is difficult to provide an adequate brief summary of the Anna O case. It is an exceptionally rich document, although it lacks descriptions of

Anna's early life and family background that would aid in putting the clinical history into a clear dynamic context.

Anna O was a 21-year-old woman from a well-to-do puritanical family. Breuer (Breuer and Freud 1893–1895/1955) describes her as showing a number of somewhat divergent personality and temperamental characteristics. She was said to have been a lively, highly intelligent, poetic, altruistic young woman whose vitality and imagination were at odds with the overall monotony of her life and the conservatism of her family. On the other hand, she was described as having periods where she was moody, labile, emotionally dramatic, willful, tenacious, and obstinate. She seemed to be at her best when caring for the weak and the needy. Even when severely disturbed, she could overcome her symptoms to help those in need.

Although she was described as "*completely unsuggestible*" (Breuer and Freud 1893–1895/1955, p. 21, their italics), she was also said to have indulged in continuous "systematic day-dreaming" which she named her "private theatre" (p. 22). In this state, she continuously "[lived] through fairy tales in her imagination" and thus detached herself from the painful monotony of her life at home. Breuer stated that "the element of sexuality was astonishingly undeveloped in her" (p. 21). At the same time, he noted her to have been "passionately fond" of her father (p. 22).

Breuer described the course of Anna O's illness as having four phases. Her problems apparently began in July 1880 after her father fell ill with a tuberculous pleuritic abscess (the period of "latent incubation"). He died on April 5, 1881. At first, Anna nursed her father intensively. Unfortunately, her own health deteriorated because of her developing nervous condition. In December 1880, she had to cease her ministrations to her father and took to her own bed ("the manifest illness").

In the first phase of illness, Anna developed "weakness, anemia . . . distaste for food . . . a typical *tussis nervosa* . . . [and] a marked craving for rest in the afternoon followed in the evening by a sleep-like state and afterwards a highly excited condition" (Breuer and Freud 1893–1895/1955, p. 23). This was "the incubation phase" that resulted in the patient's forced withdrawal from caring for her father. In December 1880, Breuer, an internist, was consulted to assess the cough. After this, he began to treat the patient intensively over the next $1\frac{1}{2}$ years, usually visiting her daily or even more frequently at times. He often spent hours at a time with Anna O, which was highly unusual for a physician at that time, especially with a hysterical patient (Freud 1925/1958; Jones 1953; Pollock 1968).

In December 1880, other symptoms appeared in Anna, including a convergent squint, left-sided occipital headache, various disturbances of vision, paresis of the front neck muscles, and contracture and anesthesia of the right upper and lower extremities, which soon extended onto the left side ("the manifest illness.")

At the beginning of treatment, Breuer (Breuer and Freud 1893–1895/1955) noted the presence in Anna of "two entirely distinct states of consciousness [which] alternated very frequently and without warning and which became more and more differentiated in the course of illness. In one of these states she recognized her surroundings; she was melancholy and anxious, but relatively normal. In the other state she hallucinated and was 'naughty'—that is to say, she was abusive, used to throw cushions . . . tore buttons off the bedclothes . . . and so on" (p. 24).

Anna reported complete amnesia for the events that took place in the naughty state and complained of "lost" time ("time-missing" in English, quoted in Ellenberger 1972; Hirschmuller 1989 reproduces a note by Anna O in English describing this and other symptoms). Small amnestic episodes ("*absences*") had already been noticed by others before this. The "disturbances invaded even her moments of relatively clear consciousness. There were extremely rapid changes of mood . . . [with] excessive high spirits and at other times severe anxiety. . . . She would complain of the profound darkness in her head, not being able to think, of becoming blind and deaf, of having two selves, a real one and an evil one which forced her to behave badly, and so on" (Breuer and Freud 1893–1895/1955, p. 24).

There were a large number of other bizarre shifting symptoms during this period. She displayed a highly complex disorganization of language ability that eventually improved when she was able to express angry feelings in words. Unfortunately, although some power of movement also returned with the improvement in speech, Anna now only spoke in English. She still understood German, however, and denied that she was speaking English.

The improvement was notable until the beginning of April, when the patient's father died. At this point, Anna had a "violent outburst of excitement . . . succeeded by profound stupor lasting about two days" (Breuer and Freud 1893–1895/1955, p. 26). Thus began the third phase of illness, the "period of persisting somnambulism" (p. 22).

In this phase, Anna experienced marked negative visual hallucinations (not seeing or recognizing people around her except for Breuer); depersonalization and derealization; an inability to understand or speak German (although retaining fluency in English, French, and Italian and speaking a pastiche of these); a change in her handedness such that she wrote left-handed with a different handwriting; anorexia (although taking food if fed by Breuer directly); and afternoon "somnolent states." After the period of somnolence, she entered "auto-hypnotic" trances in the evening.

In the period after her father's death, Anna was highly reactive to separations from Breuer. She became increasingly agitated and severely suicidal despite the intensive treatment from Breuer. Eventually this necessitated a transfer to a safer "country house" in June 1881. Subsequent research has determined that Anna was actually confined in a cottage on the grounds of a fashionable sanatorium and was attended by physicians from this hospital during Breuer's absences (Ellenberger 1970, 1972; Hirschmuller 1989). Immediately after transfer to "the country," Anna became even more wildly suicidal, agitated, and anorexic. When Breuer was unable to visit her daily, she became more and more disturbed with each day of separation.

Anna was particularly symptomatic after a separation of several weeks when Breuer took a "holiday trip" during the summer of 1881. After his return, Breuer stated he had Anna transported to Vienna for a week of intensive work on the symptoms that had surfaced during the separation.

As the patient's illness continued, the alternations of her two states of consciousness became more and more striking and discontinuous, with Anna even exhibiting apparent amnesia for periods of amnesia:

> She used to hallucinate in the middle of a conversation, run off, start climbing a tree, etc. If one caught hold of her, she would very quickly take up her interrupted sentence without knowing anything about what happened in the interval. (Breuer and Freud 1893–1895/1955, p. 31)

During this period of illness, Breuer and Anna developed the treatment method that became the foundation for psychoanalysis and dynamic psychotherapy: the "talking cure." This was characterized by "storytelling"—recital of fantasy stories often centering on the theme of a girl sitting by a sickbed. As her illness became more severe (especially after the death of her father), Anna no longer created imaginative stories while in these trances. Instead she unburdened herself of the memories, hallucinatory experiences, and imaginings that had beset her in the period between her sessions with Breuer. Breuer reported that at this point he found it necessary to use chloral hydrate and morphine to combat the agitation and psychic and physical pain in his patient when insufficient relief was provided by the talking therapy.

Anna returned to Vienna in the autumn but deteriorated markedly in December 1881—just one year after her initial decompensation. In this final phase of the illness, Breuer describes her as exhibiting a highly unusual symptom:

> Her alternating states of consciousness, which were characterized by the fact that, from morning onwards her *absences* (that is to say the emergence of her *condition seconde*) always became more frequent as the day advanced and took entire possession by the evening—these alternating states had differed from each other previously in that one (the first) was normal and the second alienated; now, however, they differed further in that in the first she lived, like the rest of us, in the winter of 1881–2, whereas in the second she lived in the winter of 1880–1, and had completely forgotten all the subsequent events. The one thing that nevertheless seemed to remain conscious most of the time was the fact that her father had died. . . . The change-over from one state to another occurred spontaneously but could also be very easily brought about by any sense impression which vividly recalled the previous year. (Breuer and Freud 1893–1895/1955, pp. 31–32)

A diary kept by Anna's mother was said by Breuer to confirm the accuracy with which Anna seemed to be living day for day in the previous year during this spontaneous age regression.

Serendipitously, Breuer discovered that Anna could relieve herself of conversion symptoms if she fully talked out the memories and emotions connected to experiences that seemed to have initially provoked the hysterical symptom. The famous method that evolved was actually a mixture of heterohypnosis induced by Breuer in the morning, with later work by Anna and Breuer together after Anna entered her daily autohypnotic state. Memories relating to specific symptoms were comprehensively and rather obsessively catalogued by Anna. The memories would then be sequentially talked out, reportedly resulting in complete disappearance of the symptom.

Anna also took control of the pace of therapy, having "formed a strong determination that the whole treatment should be finished by the anniversary of the day on which she moved to the country [June 7, 1881]" (Breuer and Freud 1893–1895/1955, p. 40). The symptom that Breuer considered "the root of her whole illness" was uncovered on this last day. This was a terrifying hallucination of a black snake coming to attack her father. She felt unable to move her arm to assist her father and hallucinated that her fingers had turned into little snakes with death's heads. She was only able to think and pray in English during this episode. Recovery of this memory was said by Breuer to have finally resolved Anna's language problems as well as most of the other conversion symptoms: "After this she left Vienna to travel for awhile but it was a considerable time before she regained her mental balance entirely. Since then she has enjoyed complete health" (p. 41).

Subsequent History of Anna O/Bertha Pappenheim

Jones (1953) in his *Life and Work of Sigmund Freud* promulgated the now-famous account of the termination of Breuer's work with Anna O. Jones states that Breuer decided to end Anna's treatment because of his wife's increasing jealousy and resentment of his overinvolvement and fascination with his attractive, charming young patient. According to Jones, on the day of termination of treatment, the patient developed a florid pseudocyesis (hysterical pregnancy). Breuer was promptly called back to the bedside. He is said to have hypnotized Anna and fled, taking his wife on a vacation to Italy, where their youngest daughter was conceived. Anna was said to have continued to be quite ill, requiring hospitalization in 1882 at "Gross Enzersdorf." She apparently became dependent on morphine. Jones also describes her as "inflam[ing] the heart" of the chief psychiatrist at the hospital. She is said to have suffered from "hallucinatory states" in the evening until at least 1887 (Jones 1953; Karpe 1961).

In a 1932 letter to Stefan Zweig, Freud (1960) recounts a similar story. He writes that Breuer was called back to Anna O's bedside on the last day of her treatment. She was "confused, writhing in abdominal cramps. Asked what was wrong with her, she replied: 'Now Dr. B's child is coming'!" (Freud 1960, p. 413). Freud criticizes Breuer for fleeing at this point—"abandon[ing] the patient"—rather than realizing the implications of the symptom. He states that the patient was hospitalized and continued to require treatment for some time after Breuer's departure. He states that one of Breuer's children confirmed this reconstruction based on a deathbed conversation with Breuer.

More Recent Historical Research

Pollock (1966, 1968, 1972, 1984) and Ellenberger (1970, 1972) and Hirschmuller (1989) have uncovered significant data about Josef Breuer and Bertha Pappenheim that sheds additional light on the Anna O case. In addition, scholarship has appeared describing Bertha Pappenheim's life and work after her return to Frankfurt in 1887 until her death in 1936 (Edinger 1968; Freeman 1972; Jensen 1970; Hirschmuller 1989; Kaplan 1984).

Although few details have been discovered about Bertha Pappenheim's early development, it is now known that she was the third child born into a prominent, conservative, and wealthy Orthodox Jewish family. There had been two other daughters in the Pappenheim family. Both died: one 4 years before Bertha's birth at age 2, and the other of consumption at the age of 17 when Bertha was 8 (Pollock 1968).

The patient's brother was born when she was $1\frac{1}{2}$ years old. Bertha was said to have never gotten along well with her brother, who was apparently less intelligent than she but who received all the educational, personal, and professional opportunities of which she was deprived in her conservative upper middle-class Jewish family (Freeman 1972).

In addition, Pollock (1968) has hypothesized that Breuer's loss of his own mother (also named Bertha) when he was 3 or 4 years old may have rendered him particularly vulnerable to strong unconscious countertransference feelings about his patient. Pollock hypothesizes that there were a number of overdetermined elements in Breuer's fascination with Anna O/Bertha P. These include "identification with her as the mourning oedipal child . . . [and] . . . revival of repressed oedipal conflicts, of repressed mourning for the dead mother, and of ambivalent feelings toward his brother" (Pollock 1968, pp. 724–725).

Ellenberger (1972) has provided fascinating historical detective work about Bertha Pappenheim. Ellenberger has documented that Bertha Pappenheim was hospitalized at the Sanatorium Bellevue in Kreuzlingen, Switzerland, from July 12 to October 29, 1882. She was hospitalized barely 1 month after the date of termination of her treatment with Breuer as reported in *Studies in Hysteria.* Ellenberger found Breuer's original detailed case summary written in 1882 as well as a follow-up note written by one of the doctors at the sanatorium. (Both are reproduced in Hirschmuller 1989). Hirschmuller (1989) documented three additional hospitalizations for "hysteria" between 1883 and 1889.

In the 1882 case summary, the patient was described as oppositional to her family's religion, although following Orthodox practices to please her father. She is described by Breuer as having difficulties with her "very serious" mother and quarreling with her brother. Breuer comments repeatedly on the patient's "truly passionate love for her father who pampered her" (Ellenberger 1972, p. 274). Breuer notes that Bertha had never been in love "to the extent that this replaced her relationship to her father" (quoted in Ellenberger 1972, p. 274).

Breuer's report also describes the exacerbation of family problems in the Pappenheim family with the illnesses of both father and daughter. Apparently, Bertha was not permitted to see her father during the last 2 months of his illness and was actually lied to about his condition even on the day of his death. She is described as being very reproachful to her mother for not permitting her an opportunity to see her father before he died. Apparently, it was Bertha's discovery of her mother's deceit about the father's death that inaugurated the period of negative hallucinations in April 1881 (Ellenberger 1972).

Breuer's 1882 case notes end in December 1881. Thus the events that led up to Anna/Bertha's hospitalization in July 1882 are not described. The later notes from the sanatorium physician describe Anna's hospitalization from July 1882 to October 1882. She was on high doses of morphine and chloral hydrate for what was thought to have been a nonhysterical facial neuralgia. She required morphine in relatively high doses even on discharge despite attempts to withdraw her from the drug.

Anna was described as showing "unpleasant irritation against her family . . . disparaging judgements against [the] ineffectiveness of science in regard to her sufferings . . . [and] . . . lack of insight into the severity of her nervous condition" (Ellenberger 1972, pp. 277–278).

She continued to be quite irritable with her mother and brother but was noted to spend "hours" under the picture of her father and talked about visiting his tomb. Her hysterical language disturbance also recurred with a loss of ability to speak German recurring in the evenings (Ellenberger 1972).

With respect to the pseudocyesis, Pollock (1968) and Ellenberger (1970, 1972) have documented that Breuer's youngest child was born on March 11, 1882, 4 months *before* Breuer's last reported last session with Anna/Bertha. If this child was a term baby she would have been conceived in June 1881, just at the time Anna/Bertha was being hospitalized and when Breuer is reported to have taken his 5-week holiday in July–August 1881 (Reeves 1982). This also was the time when Anna/Bertha was most highly symptomatic and dependent on Breuer after her father's death (e.g., only eating if fed directly by him). There is no documentation of the pseudocyesis in any of the records, although the reason for the patient's hospitalization in July 1882 has never been clarified. Breuer appears to have been unable to continue the treatment at this point.

Bertha Pappenheim's Later Life

There have been several long articles and books devoted to Bertha Pappenheim's life (Edinger 1968; Freeman 1972; Jensen 1970; Meissner 1979; Rosenbaum and Muroff 1984). It is well beyond the scope of this chapter to reproduce a full biography here. I will touch upon some of the major landmarks in her later life story in order to clarify the subsequent discussion.

Hirschmuller (1989) has uncovered the scanty extant information about Bertha Pappenheim's history during the 5 to 6 years after she left Bellevue Sanatorium in 1882. She apparently returned to Frankfurt to live with her mother. In addition to being rehospitalized several times, she studied nursing briefly. She was also encouraged to write by women friends and relatives. She wrote a series of evocative fairy tales that contained themes and images reminiscent of her hysterical hallucinations, her relationship with Breuer, and her ultimate work as a social worker (Hirschmuller 1989). The transfer of her "private theatre" to public literary works may have been particularly helpful in her overcoming her reaction to the death of her father, her hysterical illness, and the legacy of her relationship with Breuer (Hirschmuller 1989).

By 1888–1889, Pappenheim had publicly resurfaced with little overt evidence of her prior maladies. She is described as continuing "to enjoy music and her extended family and especially . . . horseback riding" (Rosenbaum 1984, p. 14) as well as becoming far more devoted to Judaism.

Pappenheim had little to do with men in her later life, although Freeman (1972) quotes Edinger as saying: "She was absolutely bewitching in a group of men. I have seen her twist men around her fingers. She must have received proposals. Even as an old woman she could be very seductive with men" (p. 209).

In 1890, Pappenheim wrote a book of stories and plays under the pseudonym of "Paul Berthold." In 1899, as P. Berthold, she wrote a three-act play called *Women's Rights,* which focused on cruel sadistic men who rape and sexually exploit women. The women were portrayed as relatively helpless but finally withholding sexual involvement from the men as punishment (Freeman 1972; Hirschmuller 1989; Meissner 1979; Rosenbaum 1984).

In 1895, Pappenheim became the directress of the Jewish Orphanage for Girls in Frankfurt, a post she held for 12 years. She became a passionate crusader for the rights of poor and oppressed women, especially in the Jewish community. She was particularly energetic in publicizing widespread prostitution and white slavery of poor Jewish women throughout Europe. She publicly battled prominent, wealthy male members of several Jewish communities who were profiting financially from these enterprises. She fearlessly travelled alone to the slums, bordellos, and brothels of Europe and the Near East in her tireless crusade to free impoverished women from sexual exploitation (Freeman 1972).

When her mother died in 1905, Pappenheim did not undergo the kind of regression that had characterized her reaction to the death of the father. However, Freeman (1972) quotes Dora Edinger, her biographer and cousin by marriage, who stated that Pappenheim's hair turned white "overnight" shortly after her mother's death.

Pappenheim was a crusader who founded several different social welfare institutions and periodicals. On the other hand, Jensen (1970) describes her as also remaining involved in the artistic and cultural milieu of bourgeois Vienna. She enjoyed beautiful furnishings and cuisine and collected lace. Jensen (1970) quotes a friend of Pappenheim a saying that "many of her acquaintances could not understand her 'double life' as a hardworking leader of social institutions and a member of the elite artistic circle" (p. 275).

At other times, however, she was perceived as stern, strict, "masculine," angry, intolerant of disagreement, given to feelings of depression and uselessness, and having periods when her "sensitivity and nervousness" surfaced (Edinger 1968; Freeman 1972; Hirschmuller 1989; Jensen 1970; Meissner 1979; Rosenbaum 1984).

She may have continued to be drawn back to her "private theatre." Jensen (1970) quotes Pappenheim as writing: "I like the word duty; for me it means a salutary and necessary counterbalance, a counterpoise to my fantasy, which is tempted to run wild and would were it not for my duties" (p. 285).

Pappenheim died of cancer in 1936 at the age of 77. She apparently remained stoically devoted to her work and intellectual pursuits despite failing health and increasing pain because of illness. Despite the stresses of her family, travels, and career, at no time during her later adult life was she ever described as having anything close to the symptoms that had plagued her during her illness in 1880–1882.

Diagnostic Formulation

As noted in the introduction, the case of Anna O/Bertha P has received numerous rediagnoses in the prior literature. In his summary of the case, Breuer himself describes Anna O as having a "dissociation of her mental personality" (Breuer and Freud 1893–1895/1955, p. 41). He goes on to note:

> It is remarkable how completely the earliest manifestation of her illness in its beginnings already exhibited its main characteristics. . . . These comprised the existence of a second state of consciousness which first emerged as a temporary *absence* and later became organized into a "*double conscience.*" (p. 42, Breuer's italics)
>
> Throughout the entire illness her two states of consciousness persisted side by side: the primary one in which she was quite normal psychically, and the secondary one which may well be likened to a dream in view of its wealth of imaginative products and hallucinations, its large gaps of memory and the lack of inhibition and control in all its associations. . . . It is hard to avoid expressing the situation by saying that the patient was split into two personalities of which one was mentally normal and the other insane. . . . Not only did the second state

> intrude into the first one, but . . . even when she was in a very bad condition—a clear-sighted and calm observer sat, as she put it, in the corner of her brain and looked on at all the mad business. (Breuer and Freud 1893–1895/1955, pp. 45–46)

DSM-III-R (American Psychiatric Association 1987) specifies the following diagnostic criteria for multiple personality disorder (MPD):

> A. The existence within the person of two or more distinct personalities or personality states (each with its own relatively enduring pattern of perceiving, relating to, and thinking about the environment and self).
>
> B. At least two of these personalities or personality states recurrently take full control of the person's behavior.

Based on the data in Breuer's case formulation, the DSM-III-R diagnostic criteria for MPD are satisfied or very close to it. One could argue that Anna O's secondary self does not fully demonstrate "an enduring pattern of . . . thinking about the environment and the self" specified by DSM-III-R to qualify for status as a full personality or personality state, because Breuer does not describe it as showing clear self-conscious awareness of itself as a separate entity. If full criteria for a personality state are not quite met, Anna O would be best conceptualized as meeting DSM-III-R criteria for dissociative disorder not otherwise specified (DDNOS). This is the diagnostic category that includes dissociative conditions just short of full-blown MPD.

Support for the MPD diagnosis is increased by comparing symptoms found in Anna O/Bertha P with those described in the literature as associated with MPD. Tables 7–1, 7–2, and 7–3 show lists of symptoms found in MPD patients. Table 7–1 compares the frequency of symptoms in three groups: a cohort of 100 MPD patients reported on in a questionnaire study (Putnam et al. 1986); a group of 38 carefully defined MPD cases found in the literature before 1960 (F. W. Putnam, unpublished data, December 1981); and 70 MPD patients reported on by Bliss (1984, 1986). Anna O/Bertha P had 12 out of 15 (80%) of the symptoms found in these patients. Table 7–2 compares Anna O/Bertha P to Bliss's cohort on a number of other symptoms. She had 6 out of 11 (54.5%) of these symptoms as well. Table 7–3 is a checklist of symptoms typical of patients with MPD and severe dissociative disorders that was developed as a teaching and research tool (Loewenstein et al.

1988). Anna O/Bertha P is described as exhibiting 26 of 39 (66.7%) of these symptoms as well (not including those listed as +/–).

Psychodynamic Data

The psychodynamic data in the case of Anna O/Bertha Pappenheim also supports a diagnosis of MPD. I will describe a number of specific psychodynamic issues in the Anna O/Bertha Pappenheim case that are identical to those that commonly recur in psychotherapeutic work with present-day MPD patients. Many of the same issues are also found in psychotherapy with child abuse survivors without MPD, although usually in less extreme forms.

Grief Reactions

Anna O/Bertha Pappenheim became acutely symptomatic with a dissociative disorder in the context of the terminal illness of her father. Putnam (1989) reports that four MPD patients in his series presented with an apparent pathological grief reaction after the death of the primary abuser, usually a parent. In my own series of MPD cases, a pathological grief reaction over the death or terminal illness of an abuser or coabuser (a nonabusing parent who gave tacit consent to or was apparently unaware of the abuse) is a common precipitant of actively symptomatic MPD or of marked symptom exacerbations in MPD patients.

A basic aspect of completion of the grief process is sufficient resolution of conflicts about the person who has died so that the bereaved can move on psychologically. However, in survivors of childhood abuse—particularly of intrafamilial sexual abuse, which is common in patients with MPD—the feelings related to the abuse and the abuser are often intensely ambivalent and divided. Frequently there is a sense of attachment, loyalty, gratification, and specialness coexisting with intense psychic pain and feelings of betrayal (Courtois 1988; Fine 1988; Gelinas 1983; Goodwin 1989; Herman 1981). There may be idealization of and identification with the abuser, fear of being anything like the abuser, loving attachment to the abuser, hatred for the abuser, terror of the abuser, loyalty to the abuser, and rationalization of the abuse and self-blame for the abuse, among many other complex feelings. In the MPD patient, these varying views of the self, the abuser, and the abuse tend to be localized in different alters (Fine 1990). Some personalities may be completely amnestic for the abuse and may have a relatively benign view of the abusive family, whereas others are in touch with traumatic memories. The grief reaction almost invariably forces greater activation of the alter personalities, just as a conflictual grief response in a person without MPD would trigger a tumult of

Table 7–1. Comparison of reported frequency of selected symptoms in studies of patients with multiple personality disorder

Symptoms	NIMH (%) (*N* = 100)	Literature Review (%) (*N* = 38)	Bliss (%) (*N* = 70)	Bertha P/ Anna O
Amnesia	98	76	75	+
Depression	88	61	84	+
Suicide attempt	68	47	79	+
Headache	66	53	43	+
Gastrointestinal symptoms	48	16	—	–
Unexplained pain	46	13	49	+/–
Psychogenic paralysis	38	32	28	+
Auditory hallucinations	29	34	50	?
Visual hallucinations	28	24	40	+
Anorexia	24	11	—	+
Visual symptoms	24	18	—	+
Anesthesias	24	24	35	+
Psychogenic deafness	16	8	—	+
Schizophrenia-like episodes	11	21	—	+
Psychogenic aphonia	10	13	—	+

Adapted from Bliss 1984; F. W. Putnam, unpublished data, December 1981; Putnam et al. 1986.

memories and powerful mixed feelings.

In addition, the death of the abuser may diminish some of the prohibition of secrecy that so often accompanies child abuse (Lister 1982). Threats of harm by abusers to prevent disclosure are common in child abuse. In MPD patients, these threats are often extremely violent or graphic, leading to profound fear of "telling the secrets" (Putnam 1989). A contemporary case illustrates these connections.

Case Study 1

Ms. A., a woman in her late 30s, was subjected to vicious physical, sexual, and emotional abuse by her cruel alcoholic father and older brother beginning at about age 4 and continuing into her adolescence. The father also abused the brother. On the other hand, the father was intellectually nurturant toward Ms. A. and encouraged her in school and in artistic pursuits. The patient reported her father would hold her head under water to reinforce his threats of retaliation if she "told." The patient's mother was cold, depressed, and remote.

Table 7–2. Comparison of symptoms reported for Bertha P/Anna O with those described by Bliss (1984) in 70 cases of multiple personality disorder

Symptoms	Bliss (%) (*N* = 70)	Bertha P/ Anna O
Nightmares	71	+/–
Rapid mood shift	69.5	+
Multiple phobias	67	+
Dazed states	66.5	+
Severe anxiety/panic	65	+
Anhedonia	62.5	–
Elimination of severe pain	60	–
Depersonalization	52	+
Derealization	52	+
Fugue states	51	–
Paranoid delusions	31	+/–

Adapted from Bliss 1984.

Ms. A. did reasonably well in her profession and as a wife and mother until the death of her father. After this she began to experience visual hallucinations, mood swings, panic attacks, poor concentration, irritability, marked psychogenic amnesia, nightmares, and flashbacks of the abuse. These were particularly intensely triggered by sexual contact with her husband. She was so continuously dissociated that she was unable to work or to perform household tasks. Her marriage deteriorated, because she often literally confused her husband with her father and brother as if she were interacting with them in a flashback. She began to abuse alcohol and pills in attempts to sleep normally and to control her symptoms. She became suicidal and engaged in self-mutilation. After a 3-year decline, Ms. A. was finally hospitalized, and the diagnosis of MPD was made. She has made slow progress since then. She still has overwhelming MPD and PTSD symptoms. The grief reaction remains an incompletely resolved problem.

Transference Themes

The concept of transference in psychotherapy is one of the most important and enduring of Freud's discoveries. According to Freud, Breuer failed to appreciate the full importance of unconscious sexual transference themes in genesis of hysterical and neurotic symptoms (Freud 1960; Jones 1953; Pollock 1968). In addition, Freud (1925/1958) notes that Breuer failed to understand and appreciate the "impersonal nature" of the transference process in his interactions with Anna/Bertha, thus missing a chance to make a discovery with far-reaching implications for psychotherapeutics.

There are a number of specific transference/countertransference problems that developed in the course of Breuer's work with Anna/Bertha that are commonly found in work with contemporary MPD patients. Although most discussions of transference in MPD have focused on the varying transference and countertransference reactions to the different alters (Wilbur 1988), in this chapter I will focus on more general transference issues that cut across alter personalities, although these may be activated in particular ways within specific alters (Loewenstein, in press).

Boundaries of the Treatment

Child abuse is fundamentally a violation of boundaries. The child's physical boundaries are breached, often in particularly cruel and intru-

Table 7–3. Symptom clusters in patients with multiple personality disorder compared with Anna O

Symptoms of MPD Patients	Anna O/ Bertha P
I. *Process Symptoms*	
1. Alter attributes (e.g. different stated age, gender, self-presentation/forms of self-expression, memory subsystems, etc.)	+
2. Passive influence symptoms/Interference phenomena	+
3. Hallucinations/Pseudohallucinations	+
4. Linguistic usage (e.g., use of 1st person plural, 3rd person singular when referring to self; use of different names for self)	–
5. Switching phenomena	+
II. *Autohypnotic Symptoms* (manifested by high hypnotizability)	
1. Spontaneous trances	+
2. Enthrallment	+
3. Spontaneous age regression	+
4. Negative hallucinations	+
5. Voluntary anesthesia	+
6. Out-of-body experiences	+
7. Trance logic	+
8. Eye-roll with switching	–
III. *Amnesia Symptoms*	
1. Blackouts/time loss	+
2. Reports of disremembered behavior	+
3. Fugues	+/–
4. Perplexing possessions	+
5. Inexplicable changes in relationships	+/–
6. Fluctuations in skills/habits/knowledge	+
7. Fragmentary recall of entire life history	–
8. Chronic mistaken identity experiences	–
9. "Micro"-dissociations	+
IV. *Somatoform Symptoms*	
1. Conversion symptoms	+
2. Pseudoseizures	–
3. Somatoform pain symptoms (e.g. headache, abdominal pain)	+
4. Somatic memory	+
5. Somatization disorder/Briquet's syndrome	?

sive ways. In addition, the appropriate boundaries between parent and child and between adults and children are also demolished. The parents of MPD patients often directly express toward their children every known sexual and aggressive impulse, which most people confine to their intrapsychic life (Fine 1988, 1990). Even while being abused, the child may be transformed into the caretaker of the adults, with a feeling of profound responsibility for the psychic integrity of the abusive parent and even of the whole family (Gelinas 1983; Herman 1981). In other ways, the MPD family may be rigidly moralistic and hierarchical, with a premium placed on maintaining an appropriate external image to the outside community (Braun and Sachs 1985).

Because the breach of boundaries was such a profound issue in the childhoods of MPD patients, it is hardly surprising that difficulties around maintenance of boundaries of the psychotherapeutic relation-

V. *PTSD Symptoms*	
1. Psychological trauma	+/–?*
2. Flashbacks/revivifications/intrusions (hyperamnesia)	+
3. Nightmares	+/–
4. Reactivity to triggers	+
5. Hyperarousal/startle response	–
6. Panic/anxiety	+
7. Numbing/avoidance/detachment	–
VI. *Affective Symptoms*	
1. Depressed mood (differentiate between mood disorder localized in specific alter(s) versus across "total human being")	+
2. Hypomania/mood swings (differentiate between mood disorder localized in specific alter(s) versus "total human being"; mood swings not due to interference phenomena between alters)	+
3. Vegetative symptoms (must be differentiated from PTSD symptoms; e.g., middle of night awakening due to nightmares, etc.)	+
4. Suicidal thoughts/attempts/self-mutilation	+
5. Guilt	–
6. Helpless/hopeless	+/–

* The death of her father was traumatic to Anna O but would not have met DSM-III-R criteria.

Adapted from Loewenstein et al. 1988.

ship play a powerful role in the transference of these patients (Fine 1989, 1990; Loewenstein, in press). Virtually every treatment of an MPD patient will have recurrent themes of the testing of boundaries, often in exceptionally creative ways. Although therapeutic flexibility is very important in the successful treatment of MPD patients, assiduous interpretive attention to the boundaries and the frame of the treatment is critical for a good outcome (Greaves 1988; Loewenstein, in press). This is one of the recurrent paradoxes in the treatment of MPD patients.

In addition, MPD patients are victimized in adulthood more frequently than control populations (Coons and Milstein 1986). MPD patients commonly give histories of sexual involvement (often recurrent) with teachers, ministers, and psychotherapists. MPD patients usually harbor intense mistrust for caretakers based on these abusive experiences, but they also seem naively vulnerable to repeated exploitation. MPD patients frequently find their way into actual or symbolic recreations of the childhood abuse experience with an exploitative therapist or one with unresolved characterologic or countertransference problems (Kluft 1989a, 1989b).

In this way, MPD patients often become involved in psychotherapeutic relationships that, although not strictly sexualized, are characterized by major alterations in the typical boundaries of treatment, often with an unconsciously eroticized quality. The problems related to these situations are so stereotyped and so frequent that much of the consultation practice of the community of MPD experts is devoted to disentangling patients and therapists from these disastrous situations (Greaves 1988; Kluft 1989a, 1989b; Marmer 1991). Additionally, in many stalemated MPD treatments, more subtle boundary problems can be detected.

It is beyond the scope of this chapter to explicate completely the reasons for this recurrent transference/countertransference pattern. However, even relatively skilled and experienced therapists can become enveloped in the powerful projections and projective identifications of the MPD patient. It may be that the intense ongoing dissociation by the MPD patient in therapy leads to a kind of mutual dissociation of the reality implications of the loss of treatment boundaries. A kind of unconscious shared dissociation ensues in which the therapist seems to forget all that he or she knew before about therapy and the patient ignores the danger signals heralding another interpersonal disaster.

The patient's powerful projected wishes accompanied by a kind of trance logic (hypnotically induced toleration of logical inconsistency) (Bliss 1980; Orne 1959) leave the therapist seemingly less able to resist impulses recognized as inappropriate in other therapy contexts. This is often accompanied by rationalization of these deviations as necessary and therapeutic. Therapists who have insufficiently worked through a variety of countertransference issues (e.g., rescue fantasies and need for narcissistic gratification from patients) will be more vulnerable to such difficulties.

I do not wish to appear to support the typical MPD patient's abuse-related cognition that it is the patient's "fault" that these treatments go awry. This reaction is actually a part of the unconscious repetition inherent in the development of these transference disasters: the victim blaming him- or herself for causing the abuse. It is important to emphasize that the therapist is the professional in the treatment and thus bears the full responsibility for the clinical judgments that are made, for good or for ill.

Experienced therapists generally become much more inured to the dissociative therapeutic field engendered by the MPD patient. Neophyte therapists often do better with MPD patients if the potential problems around boundaries and their significance are discussed very early in consultation or supervision. Nonetheless, it is important to emphasize that the specific transference/countertransference problems around boundary management are an inherent aspect of the treatment of MPD patients that lasts the length of the therapy. Clinicians should expect these problems to recur continually (Fine 1989; Loewenstein, in press).

Overinvolvement, intense fascination, and assumption of responsibility for all aspects of the MPD patient's life is a recurrent countertransference problem for vulnerable or unsophisticated therapists with MPD patients. In many cases, the overinvolvement becomes more and more consuming until, like Breuer, the therapist is finally forced to withdraw, usually precipitously. When this occurs, the patient reacts with intense despair, confusion, and grief. There is an increase in the patient's sense of mistrust and betrayal over another relationship that should have been nurturant and helpful but instead is injurious and hurtful. Subsequent psychotherapy becomes far more difficult because of the increased conflict over formation of a therapeutic alliance with the new therapist.

In this situation, the therapist is also frequently devastated by the realization of the true dimensions of the problems in the treatment. He or she often feels extremely guilty, inadequate, and ashamed at what has occurred, especially over having hurt the patient so deeply. The therapist may question his or her ability to work with patients at all. It is often advisable for therapists to reenter psychotherapy themselves at these times to understand, as Breuer never could, the specific unconscious forces that have led to this countertransference disaster. If the therapist continues in work with MPD patients, it is vital that he or she also obtain ongoing consultation and supervision to help with reactions to the previous difficulties.

The next case study illustrates these issues. A multitude of additional examples could be provided.

Case Study 2

Ms. B. is a woman in her 40s who was diagnosed with MPD by a very senior psychiatrist without prior experience with MPD. As the MPD unfolded, Ms. B.'s numerous child personalities emerged. She became massively suicidal and dependent, calling her doctor and demanding more and more therapy time. The psychiatrist became increasingly preoccupied with her, talked of nothing else, and neglected his relationship with his wife and children. Eventually he saw Ms. B. more and more frequently, often staying with her for 6 to 7 hours a day. At various points, he personally chauffeured her to the hospital. As he expanded his contact with the patient, she became even more suicidal and controlling.

Treatment was finally ended because of the toll the therapy was taking on the therapist's life, income, and family situation. There was a massive crisis, suicide attempts, and an emergency hospitalization of Ms. B. Eventually she was transferred to a hospital in another city. She experienced the termination as a profound abandonment in which she was banished because of her badness.

The psychiatrist was completely demoralized by the experience, his clinical confidence badly shattered. His marriage and family life also were troubled for some time after the termination of the case. The psychiatrist reentered psychotherapy and appeared to work through the crisis.

At the new hospital, another psychiatrist assumed Ms. B.'s care. Although the overall treatment frame has improved, the second psychiatrist also has had difficulties in managing a large number of issues relating to boundaries and limits in her treatment. Ms. B. remains quite regressed, overwhelmed by traumatic memories, and exhibits a large number of warring alters.

Several other transference themes also occur in the case of Anna/Bertha that are similar to those found in contemporary MPD cases. For example, MPD patients usually have profound difficulties around feelings of loss of control in therapy and in their lives. Difficulties around control in MPD patients have many determinants, including reactions to amnesia, switching, anxiety over emergence or dominance by other alters, intrusion of traumatic memories, and concerns about vulnerability and dependency on the therapist. The latter may be especially evoked at times of separation from the therapist. MPD patients frequently try to handle this by attempting to direct and orchestrate their treatment in various ways.

For example, Anna O set a termination date in her treatment that coincided almost exactly with the date in the previous year when she had been forced by Breuer to move away from him into the country (surely a case of "You can't fire me! I quit!"). This was also the time when Breuer left on a 5-week vacation, during which his wife conceived their youngest child. At a deeper level, Anna/Bertha was probably attempting to undo her feeling of loss of control and helplessness at her father's abandonment of her through his death.

However, frequently these situations have an unconscious traumatic context as well. For example, an MPD patient repeatedly called her therapist on weekends in various crises, seemingly unable to tolerate the separation from him. Eventually it was learned that weekends were the times in her childhood when she had been most likely to be left by her mother to stay alone with her father, who had severely abused her. Clarification of this and work with several personalities connected to the weekend abuse from the patient's childhood led to a significant diminution in the calls. More typical interpretations directed at the patient's apparent hostile dependency had seemed only to worsen the problem.

Bertha Pappenheim's Later Life and the MPD Diagnosis

Recent psychoanalytic interpretations of Bertha Pappenheim's later life and career have focussed on her hypothesized unresolved oedipal feelings for her beloved father (Meissner 1979; Freeman 1972). Others have posited pre-oedipal disturbances related to depression and withdrawal by her mother after the death of Pappenheim's siblings and the birth of her brother (Gargiulo 1984; Meissner 1979; Pollock 1968).

Meissner (1979) and Freeman (1972) strongly suggest that Pappenheim's unresolved oedipal disappointments with her father and Breuer were a major unconscious determinant of her lifelong crusade to help sexually exploited Jewish women and to battle Jewish businessmen profiting from prostitution and the white slave trade. Freeman (1972) even suggests that Pappenheim had unconscious prostitution fantasies related to her unresolved oedipal incestuous wishes.

However, no one has considered whether Pappenheim was actually sexually abused in childhood, struggling throughout her life with memories of actual incestuous experiences and not with incestuous fantasies. As the preceding discussion suggests, the historical, phenomenological, and psychodynamic data are completely consistent with the hypothesis that Bertha Pappenheim was subjected to some form of childhood sexual abuse.

The simplest formulation would be that Pappenheim was sexually abused by her father. This would most parsimoniously explain her intense transference reaction to Breuer. It would also represent a more satisfactory and less patronizing way of understanding Pappenheim's passionate involvement with the white slavery problem in the Jewish community. This notion would also be consistent with Pollock's (1968) idea that Pappenheim's mother was depressed and unavailable during her early childhood, leaving her to more intense involvements with her father.

Freeman (1972) suggests that Anna/Bertha's second "bad" self contained unacceptable sexual fantasies and wishes. This secondary self also might have contained unacceptable memories of childhood sexual experiences. At the same time, the host personality idealized and worshiped her father.

Based on Pappenheim's later fictional work, one might also speculate that Pappenheim was not only abused by her father but also witnessed or knew of her father's sexual exploitation or involvement with other women. This might have increased her vulnerability to fears of abandonment after an actual or symbolic seduction.

Freeman (1972) suggests that Anna/Bertha may have been sexually stimulated by her father while nursing him, increasing the pressure of her unacceptable oedipal wishes. Another way to understand the roots of Anna/Bertha's breakdown into florid dissociative pathology is the supposition that the original sexual abuse occurred with a more distant relative or with servants employed by the family. The parents would then be failed protectors who should have been aware of the abuse and its consequences but were not directly involved in major abusive acts. MPD patients often have powerful loving and idealizing feelings for neglectful, coabusive parents who fail to prevent abuse by others. The negative feelings toward such parents are often very difficult to get at in therapy and are a source of profound pain for MPD patients.

In either scenario, we can hypothesize that Anna/Bertha's father, sick and regressed, behaved in ways during his terminal illness that triggered dissociated sexual memories in his daughter. This shattered her idealization of him as well as flooding her with intrusions of dissociated memories of earlier abuse.

This hypothesis that Bertha Pappenheim was abused outside of her immediate family might also help to explain her symptomatic recovery and relative psychological stability throughout her later life. Kluft (1985) has described the natural history of MPD over the life cycle. He notes that a subset of MPD patients are relatively asymptomatic or psychologically compensated throughout much of their lives, whereas others are more continually troubled (Kluft 1991). Kluft has also suggested that MPD patients with relatively circumscribed periods of abuse in childhood may be more likely to describe asymptomatic or latent MPD life histories punctuated by symptomatic episodes (R. P. Kluft, personal communication, April 1985).

In this formulation, Bertha Pappenheim was able to resolve sufficiently her grief reaction over her father because he was not her primary abuser. She could eventually reinvest in her family and involve herself in her father's religion. Perhaps she was able to discuss her abuse experiences with her mother or another woman, allowing some relief and diminution of pain, guilt, and despair. This might explain her solid attachment to her mother in later life and her bonding with women in her subsequent work. At the same time, her disappointment in her father over his sexual indiscretions and/or his failure to protect her from another abuser (perhaps a member of another prominent family) would fuel her lifelong crusade against sexual exploitation of women by more powerful and sexually rapacious men. With the slow recovery from her breakdown, her multiplicity sealed over. It reemerged in a subtle fashion: in her nightmare reveries, in her temperamental shifts, in her uncanny ability to bewitch men, and in her divergent tastes and habits.

Shortly after her reemergence as a social worker in Frankfurt, the psychoanalytic movement dissociated hypnosis, dissociation, child abuse, and an interest in severe psychological trauma. It is only now that we are beginning to fully appreciate the legacy of Bertha Pappenheim.

References

American Psychiatric Association: Diagnostic and Statistical Manual of Mental Disorders, 3rd Edition, Revised. Washington, DC, American Psychiatric Association, 1987

Armbruster RA: Personality characteristics of contemporary American female social workers as compared to those of Bertha Pappenheim (Anna O.). Dissertation Abstracts 43(1-B):229, 1982

Bliss E: Multiple personalities: a report of 14 cases with implications for schizophrenia and hysteria. Arch Gen Psychiatry 37:1388–1397, 1980

Bliss EL: A symptom profile of patients with multiple personalities including MMPI results. J Nerv Ment Dis 172:197–202, 1984

Bliss EL: Multiple Personality, Allied Disorders and Hypnosis. New York, Oxford University Press, 1986

Bloch DA: The family therapy of Anna O.: other times, other paradigms, in Anna O.: Fourteen Contemporary Reinterpretations. Edited by Rosenbaum M, Muroff M. New York, Free Press, 1984, pp 141–148

Bolkosky S: The alpha and omega of psychoanalysis: reflections on Anna O. and Freud's Vienna. Psychoanal Rev 69(1):131–150, 1982

Braun BG, Sachs RG: The development of multiple personality disorder: predisposing, precipitating, and perpetuating factors, in Childhood Antecedents of Multiple Personality. Edited by Kluft RP. Washington, DC, American Psychiatric Press, 1985, pp 37–64

Breuer J, Freud S: Studies on Hysteria (1893–1895), in The Standard Edition of the Complete Psychological Works of Sigmund Freud, Vol 2. Translated and edited by Strachey J. London, Hogarth Press, 1955

Coons PM, Milstein V: Psychosexual disturbances in multiple personality: characteristics, etiology, treatment. J Clin Psychiatry 47:106–110, 1986

Courtois C: Healing the Incest Wound: Adult Survivors in Therapy. New York, WW Norton, 1988

Edinger D: Bertha Pappenheim: Freud's Anna O. Highland Park, IL, Congregation Solel, 1968

Ellenberger HF: The Discovery of the Unconscious: The History and Evolution of Dynamic Psychiatry. New York, Basic Books, 1970

Ellenberger HF: The story of Anna O: a critical review with new data. J Hist Behav Sci 8:267–279, 1972

Fine CG: Thoughts on the cognitive perceptual substrates of multiple personality disorder. Dissociation 1(4):5–9, 1988

Fine CG: Treatment errors and iatrogenesis across therapeutic modalities in MPD and allied dissociative disorders. Dissociation 2(2):77–82, 1989

Fine CG: The cognitive sequelae of incest, in Incest-Related Disorders of Adult Psychopathology. Edited by Kluft RP. Washington, DC, American Psychiatric Press, 1990, pp 161–182

Freeman L: The Story of Anna O. New York, Walker, 1972

Freud S: Psychotherapy of hysteria (1895), in The Standard Edition of the Complete Psychological Works of Sigmund Freud, Vol 2. Edited by Strachey J. London, Hogarth Press, 1955a, pp 253–305

Freud S: Five lectures on psycho-analysis (1910), in The Standard Edition of the Complete Psychological Works of Sigmund Freud, Vol 11. Edited by Strachey J. London, Hogarth Press, 1955b, pp 9–55

Freud S: An autobiographical study (1925), in The Standard Edition of the Complete Psychological Works of Sigmund Freud, Vol 20. Translated and Edited by Strachey J. London, Hogarth Press, 1958, pp 7–70

Freud S: Letters of Sigmund Freud. Selected and edited by Freud E. New York, Basic Books, 1960, pp 412–413

Gargiulo G: Anna O.: an English object relations approach, in Anna O.: Fourteen Contemporary Reinterpretations. Edited by Rosenbaum M, Muroff M. New York, Free Press, 1984, pp 149–160

Gelinas DJ: The persisting negative effects of incest. Psychiatry 46:312–332, 1983

Goodwin J: Sexual Abuse: Incest Victims and Their Families, 2nd Edition. Chicago, IL, Year Book Medical, 1989

Goshen C: The original case material of psychoanalysis. Am J Psychiatry 108:829–834, 1952

Greaves G: Common errors in the treatment of multiple personality disorder. Dissociation 1:61–66, 1988

Herman J: Father-Daughter Incest. Cambridge, MA, Harvard University Press, 1981

Hirschmuller A: The Life and Work of Josef Breuer: Physiology and Psychoanalysis. New York, New York University Press, 1989

Hurst LC: What was wrong with Anna O. J R Soc Med 75:129–131, 1982

Jensen EM: Anna O—a study of her later life. Psychoanal Q 39:269–293, 1970

Jones E: The Life and Work of Sigmund Freud (3 Vols). New York, Basic Books, 1953

Kaplan M: Anna O. and Bertha Pappenheim: an historical perspective, in Anna O.: Fourteen Contemporary Reinterpretations. Edited by Rosenbaum M, Muroff M. New York, Free Press, 1984, pp 101–117

Karpe R: The rescue complex in Anna O's final identity. Psychoanal Q 30:1–27, 1961

Kluft R (ed): Childhood Antecedents of Multiple Personality. Washington, DC, American Psychiatric Press, 1985

Kluft RP: Unsuspected multiple personality disorder: an uncommon source of protracted resistance, interruption, and failure in psychoanalysis. Hillside J Clin Psychiatry 9:100–115, 1987

Kluft RP: The rehabilitation of therapists overwhelmed by their work with multiple personality disordered patients. Dissociation 2:244–249, 1989a

Kluft RP: Treating the patient who has been sexually exploited by a previous therapist. Psychiatr Clin North Am 12:483–500, 1989b

Kluft RP: Clinical presentations of multiple personality disorder. Psychiatr Clin North Am 14:605–629, 1991

Lister E: Forced silence: a neglected dimension of trauma. Am J Psychiatry 139:872–876, 1982

Loewenstein RJ: Posttraumatic and dissociative aspects of transference and countertransference in the treatment of multiple personality disorder, in Clinical Perspectives on Multiple Personality Disorder. Edited by Kluft RP, Fine CG. Washington, DC, American Psychiatric Press (in press)

Loewenstein RJ, Hornstein N, Farber B: Open trial of clonazepam in the treatment of posttraumatic stress symptoms in MPD. Dissociation 1(3):3–12, 1988

Macmillan M: The cathartic method and the expectancies of Breuer and Anna O. Int J Clin Exp Hypn 25:106–119, 1977

Marmer S: Multiple personality disorder: a psychoanalytic perspective. Psychiatr Clin North Am 14:677–693, 1991

Martorano J: The psychopharmacological treatment of Anna O., in Anna O.: Fourteen Contemporary Reinterpretations. Edited by Rosenbaum M, Muroff M. New York, Free Press, 1984, pp 85–100

Meissner W: A study on hysteria: Anna O rediviva. Annals of Psychoanalysis 7:17–52, 1979

Muroff M: Anna O: psychoanalysis and group process therapy, in Anna O.: Fourteen Contemporary Reinterpretations. Edited by Rosenbaum M, Muroff M. New York, Free Press, 1984, pp 71–84

Nakdimen KA: Psychoanalysis and multiple personality. Am J Psychiatry 145:896–897, 1988

Orne MT: The nature of hypnosis: artifact and essence. Journal of Abnormal and Social Psychology 58:277–299, 1959

Orr-Andrawes A: The case of Anna O: a neuropsychiatric perspective. J Am Psychoanal Assoc 35:387–419, 1987

Pollock G: Mourning and childhood loss: their possible significance in the Josef Breuer-Bertha Pappenheim relationship. Bulletin of the Association of Psychoanalytic Medicine 5:51–54, 1966

Pollock GH: The possible significance of childhood object loss in the Josef Breuer-Bertha Pappenheim (Anna O)-Sigmund Freud relationship. J Am Psychoanal Assoc 16:711–739, 1968

Pollock G: Bertha Pappenheim's pathological mourning: possible effects of early sibling loss. J Am Psychoanal Assoc 20:476–493, 1972

Pollock GH: Anna O.: Insight, hindsight, and foresight, in Anna O.: Fourteen Contemporary Reinterpretations. Edited by Rosenbaum M, Muroff M. New York, Free Press, 1984, pp 26–33

Putnam F: Diagnosis and Treatment of Multiple Personality Disorder. New York, Guilford, 1989

Putnam FW, Guroff JJ, Silberman EK, et al: The clinical phenomenology of multiple personality disorder: 100 recent cases. J Clin Psychiatry 47:285–293, 1986

Reeves C: Breuer, Freud, and the case of Anna O: a re-examination. Journal of Child Psychotherapy 8:203–214, 1982

Reichard S: A re-examination of "Studies in Hysteria." Psychoanal Q 25:155-177, 1956

Rosenbaum M: Anna O. (Bertha Pappenheim): her history, in Anna O.: Fourteen Contemporary Reinterpretations. Edited by Rosenbaum M, Muroff M. New York, Free Press, 1984, pp 1–26

Rosenbaum M, Muroff M (eds): Anna O.: Fourteen Contemporary Reinterpretations. New York, Free Press, 1984

Spiegel JP: The case of Anna O: cultural aspects, in Anna O.: Fourteen Contemporary Reinterpretations. Edited by Rosenbaum M, Muroff M. New York, Free Press, 1984, pp 52–58

Spotnitz H: The case of Anna O: aggression and the narcissistic countertransference, in Anna O.: Fourteen Contemporary Reinterpretations. Edited by Rosenbaum M, Muroff M. New York, Free Press, 1984, pp 132–140

Steinmann A: Anna O.: female, 1880–1882; Bertha Pappenheim: female, 1980–1982, in Anna O.: Fourteen Contemporary Reinterpretations. Edited by Rosenbaum M, Muroff M. New York, Free Press, 1984, pp 118–131

Wilbur C: Multiple personality disorder and transference. Dissociation 1:73–76, 1988

Chapter 8

The Dora Syndrome: Attempts to Restructure Childhood in Adult Victims of Child Abuse

Kathryn C. Krieg, M.D.
Jean M. Goodwin, M.D., M.P.H.

My (K. K.) first year as a psychiatric resident taught much about descriptive psychiatric and medical diagnosis, taking care of sick people, and holding up my end of a doctor-patient relationship. Useful as this was, it did not prepare me for the 8 young adult victims of child abuse who appeared in the 27-patient caseload I acquired in my second year of training. In these patients, diagnoses were multiple and shifting; and diagnoses offered little refuge from the Alice-in-Wonderland confusions of a doctor-patient relationship that sometimes, like the Cheshire cat, disappeared entirely. Yet all of the patients seemed to have a strong desire for psychotherapeutic treatment, which they pursued at great cost and sacrifice.

My initial confusion and frustration in these cases seemed an echo of Freud's "cri de coeur" at the end of his report on the Dora case (1905/1971): "I do not know what kind of help she wanted from me" (p. 144). Freud, too, struggled with his patient's paradoxical desire for treatment in the face of fierce resistance to it. When, after quitting treatment on 1 hour's notice, Dora applied to Freud (on April Fool's Day) to return to treatment, he could only conclude, "She was not in earnest over her request" (p. 143).

Recent reinterpretations of the Dora case (Erikson 1962; Jennings 1986; Krohn and Krohn 1982; Mai 1985; Malcolm 1987; Marcus 1985; Sprengnether 1985) have emphasized Dora's hurt and anger at the emotional abuse that so overshadowed her childhood. Her mother, described by Freud as having a "housewife's psychosis," was somatically preoccupied with the gonorrhea she had contracted from her husband, and if she was not psychotic, she was at least peculiar.

Her father, syphilitic secondary to his compulsive philandering and also seriously consumptive, was attempting to turn over the teenaged Dora to the husband of his current mistress. Although Freud wanted Dora to explore her own angry and sexual wishes toward parents and parent figures, Dora wanted something else. She wanted her father to give up his mistress, Frau K. Dora wanted an acknowledgement of and apology for the shabby way that she herself had been used in the affair. This she eventually extracted from the mistress and the supernumerary husband, if not from her parents. Dora had dreams about a young suitor who later did come forward to marry her, thus proving that her hopes for a normal life had not been entirely destroyed by her parents' failures. She was also trying to improve herself by attending lectures and through other academic pursuits. Finally, she wanted help with her anger at her parents, which had emerged as self-defeating somatic complaints—inability to walk, difficulty swallowing, abdominal pain, cough, vaginal discharge, migraine, aphonia, pseudoseizures, difficulty breathing, and facial pain. These were not resolved in treatment. When Felix Deutsch (1957) saw Dora 24 years after treatment, she was complaining of vertigo and insomnia and her physician described her as "one of the most repulsive hysterics" (p. 167) he had ever met.

In working with the eight adult victims of child abuse in my own training caseload, I found that, as has been suggested in the Dora case, the picture was clarified if I put the abusive childhood at the center of the clinical work. Child abuse in these cases was less subtle than in the Dora case, involving physical attacks in all eight patients and paternal sexual abuse in four. Two cases had been investigated by child protective services. In all, there was evidence of some attempt to reform or reconstruct the defective abusive parents. The only patient not still actively engaged with parents had lost both to death. In all patients, too, there was an active attempt to restore and restructure childhood deficits in adulthood and to complete adolescent tasks. College and education were the typical focus of these attempts. Only two of the eight patients had managed to stay clear of an educational institution for more than a year before entering treatment; on follow-up, one of those has returned to school already, and the second was planning to return. The universal noncompliance with treatment seen in these patients became easier to tolerate when connected with their rage at and wariness of the sadistic parent that they expected would resurface in the therapist.

In this discussion, we will explore one case in detail and use examples from all eight to illustrate how focusing on the child abuse experience illuminates all four aspects of what we have called the Dora syndrome:

1. The inability to comply with the rules of treatment;
2. The attempt to reform and reconstruct abusive parents;
3. The attempt in adulthood to restore and restructure childhood deficits; and
4. The struggle to recognize and understand chronic rage that has been expressed previously only self-destructively.

The Patient Population

The 8 patients who found their way into my (K. K.) training caseload included 7 women and 1 man, aged 22 to 38. Their demographics resembled those of adolescence much more than of young adulthood. None was living with a spouse; only three had children, and only two of those were living with the child. Five of the eight were in school; the other three were either recently graduated or planning to return to college.

Substance abuse, eating disorders, and violence toward self and others were common symptoms in this group. Two had made suicide attempts; one physically abused her own children; and one has had problems with physical fights in adulthood. Three had severe substance abuse problems, and two had been diagnosed as having eating disorders. Only two are free of all three behavioral problems.

Extensive compliance problems were present in these patients. Five were veterans of prior therapy; in four of these five cases, compliance problems were noted by a previous therapist. Inappropriate hypersexual behavior was a problem in three of those cases; two of those three were incest victims. "Not taking therapy seriously" was noted in two cases and frequent missed appointments in two cases.

In the present course of therapy, all actively avoided the therapeutic process. Four missed appointments frequently. This of course is a universal issue in psychotherapy, but in these patients the problem was extreme. One patient missed the next five sessions after her therapist "made" her cry. With three patients there was chronic confusion about the appointment times; as a result, the patients would come on the wrong day or at the wrong hour or repeatedly believe a session to be canceled when it was not. The dynamics were clear with one patient who worked out a very intermittent schedule of appointments because "it's too depressing to talk about these things"; after sessions she would cry and feel disorganized for days. Other avoidance strategies used by these patients included sleeping in sessions, requesting that it be the therapist who did the talking in sessions, and refusing to discuss major issues like suicidality.

The following is a more detailed report of one of the eight cases. It illustrates the themes of noncompliance with rules of treatment, attempted reconstructions of parents and childhood, and the struggle with chronic hostility.

The Case of Betty

Betty is a 28-year-old single woman, a university student, who was beginning her fifth year of therapy with her fourth therapist at the time I met her. Transfer summaries from my 3 predecessors quoted her chief complaint as "I need someone to talk to." She also said that she needed help dealing with severe and often overwhelming anger.

Previous therapists had noted her inability to comply with the structure of psychotherapy. She frequently missed appointments or came late, even though a fee was assessed for this and her finances were limited. However, she did not tolerate any appointments missed by the therapist and at one point took her then-therapist's name plate and kept it during his illness and for several weeks after.

Betty was often described as "silly" and "giggly." Therapists commented that she did not take her therapy sessions seriously. Her second therapist noted that she developed an intense erotic transference in therapy and felt that this was the only reason she continued to attend sessions at all.

In addition, Betty was described as sexually promiscuous, maintaining relationships with five different men at the time of her transfer to my caseload. A previous therapist thought that her boyfriends number four and five might be enacted representations of departing therapists two and three. Betty's known background was that the patient's mother had left the family when Betty was 2 years old, leaving Betty and her three brothers in the care of their father. From ages 2 through 13, Betty lived with her father. At age 13, she was placed in foster care, presumably because of her father's bankruptcy, where she remained until adulthood.

Betty began our first session by announcing that she had finally "discovered" the nature of her problem with her previous therapist and that she hoped that with continued therapy she could decide what to do about it. The "problem" as she saw it was that she was unhappy and exhausted from her efforts to maintain relationships with five boyfriends but frightened about changing this because of her fear of being alone, particularly at night. This reminded her of lonely nights spent in numerous foster homes; this in turn led to the story of how Betty came to be placed in foster care in the first place. Over the next three sessions, she began to describe her father's cruel physical abuse of her.

Betty described her father as cruel and unpredictable. The most frightening aspect of her abuse was that she never knew when to expect it. She noted that her father hit her with whatever was available—tools, lumber, and even a baseball bat—and that she was always bruised as a child. On one occasion, her father had held her face under water in the toilet and she had feared death by drowning.

Betty failed to attend our fourth session without notice—my first encounter with her noncompliance. She began the next session by asking me if I was angry with her—a question I was to hear often as Betty looked for evidence in me of the cruel sadistic authority figure she had learned to expect in childhood. She then observed that if her therapist "hit a nerve" in a session, it generally led to her missing the next appointment. She said that her missing was not deliberate and that she felt sad when she realized what had happened. It was clear in this situation that we had "hit a nerve" in those early sessions about her father. We began using this metaphor to examine each session before it ended in order to note where we may have "hit a nerve" and to anticipate difficulties getting to the next appointment.

Spending the last 5 minutes of each session in this kind of review improved compliance. Betty often attended as many as six consecutive sessions, a new record for her.

Nonetheless, a pattern of occasionally missed sessions continued as well as chronic lateness for appointments. Any lingering doubts I had that Betty's noncompliance was the simple result of lack of motivation for psychotherapeutic treatment were dispelled one cold winter morning when Betty rushed into the clinic 15 minutes late for her appointment. Following her apology, she told me that she had taken a taxicab 12 miles to the clinic; the cost was double that of her fee.

In our second month of therapy, Betty began planning to visit her mother. It was then that I became aware of her extensive efforts to reform and reconstruct the mother who abandoned her at age 2. At age 15, Betty had researched her mother's whereabouts with clues from a relative. She arranged a train trip and presented herself at her mother's home. She invited her mother to a "family reunion" (minus father) that year and since then has maintained contact through letters, telephone calls, and yearly visits. She has gone to great lengths to establish this relationship and to learn more about her mother.

Upon her return from this visit, Betty had two major concerns. She noted that her mother had gained weight and thought that if she had the opportunity to live with her mother, she would have been able to structure a program of diet and exercise and "get her in shape." Betty will have an opportunity to do this in her chosen career. She is studying physical therapy in college and hopes to help people "get in shape."

Second, Betty wondered why she had not yet been invited to spend Christmas with her mother. She then reflected back to the many past Christmases spent alone and began to make plans in anticipation of another lonely holiday. However, early in our fifth month of therapy, Betty announced excitedly in a session that she had been invited to spend her first Christmas ever with her mother. From then until Christmas, much time in our sessions was spent on anticipation of this occasion. One focus was on choosing the "perfect gift" for each participant in the celebration. Betty was so concerned with Christmas being "done right" that we even discussed etiquette rules of gift-giving and receiving.

It was during this preholiday period that I learned Betty had been taking herself to see the *Nutcracker* ballet each year at Christmas time for the past 10 years. She had effectively established her own holiday tradition in the absence of parents who might normally do this.

I learned also of the significance of ballet in Betty's life. Her excitement in anticipation of spending Christmas with her mother was surpassed only by her excitement that a new semester would bring her the opportunity to take the ballet classes for which she had been waiting for 20 years. She described her childhood dreams of becoming a ballerina and her desperate wish for lessons. She participated avidly in her ballet class and devoted much time to practice.

We were in our seventh month of therapy before Betty discussed the problems with anger and hostility that had first brought her to psychotherapy years before. A former woman friend had stolen her collection of pennies. Her anger at this was so overwhelming that it resulted in a violent physical attack on the woman, as well as a near-fatal attack on the woman's cat. She described a few other such episodes of overwhelming rage and noted that all episodes had in common a loss of memory for some of her actions.

I was intrigued and puzzled as to how this presumed theft of a penny collection could trigger so much anger. I soon learned that the pennies were a link to an important childhood memory of a past Christmas. Betty and her brothers learned that they were to be together with their father on Christmas. In their efforts to purchase the "perfect gift" for their father, the four children pooled their respective penny collections and were able to afford one of their father's favorite brands of tobacco.

An ongoing theme in Betty's life was an avid interest and participation in competitive sports. She joined teams for softball and basketball, studied dance and gymnastics in school, and trained strenuously for marathon races. As I pondered the importance of athletics in Betty's life, I learned that her father had been very proud of these achievements. According to Betty, he had proudly displayed her awards and bragged to friends and relatives. In fact, Betty's refusal to participate in basketball one year resulted in a public beating, which led to the involvement of Protective Services and the dissolution of Betty's family. Betty's athletic accomplishments seemed a means to gain the approval of a father reconstructed from the few pleasant memories of him that remained.

As we worked on this material from childhood, Betty's problem of the five boyfriends she had needed to assuage her loneliness began to resolve itself. One of the five boyfriends had seemed different from the beginning. She agonized about setting limits on her contact with the other four men, worrying and feeling guilty about how much they would be hurt. It seemed clear that Betty did not wish to see herself as someone who abandoned others in the way her mother had abandoned her. Betty has put a great deal of effort into maintaining friendships with these former boyfriends. An ongoing issue has been Betty's struggle to explain to her current boyfriend the importance of these friendships. At first, I struggled along with Betty, trying to understand the almost desperate manner in which she pursued these friendships. As I learned more about the depth of Betty's pain over the loss of her family, it seemed clear that these former boyfriends were part of Betty's reconstructed family. They represent her lost brothers. It was no longer surprising that she clung to them so stubbornly.

As Betty transitioned from five boyfriends to one, her fear of being alone evolved into an active seeking out of solitude. At first she described spending her time alone studying and doing housework. Only later did Betty describe in an almost defiant manner her enjoyment of watching children's television programs and finger painting. Once again, she was making attempts to restructure her childhood—this time, Betty is so quiet and so good at amusing herself that mother couldn't possibly want to leave.

Although attendance at sessions was no longer a crippling problem after the first 6 months, Betty found other means of escaping the pain of treatment. On one occasion she took diphenhydramine (Benadryl) prior to coming which resulted in her falling asleep during the session. These and other episodes of noncompliance were much easier to understand (and to tolerate) within the framework of making the childhood abuse the central focus of our therapy. She continued to try to shield me from her neediness and grief so she would not be abandoned, and from her anger, so she would not be berated and beaten.

Discussion

Putting the Abusive Childhood at the Center of the Clinical Work

Freud noted how concerned Dora was about setting the historical record straight (1905/1971). He wrote that she seemed "almost beside herself at the idea . . . that she had merely fancied the conditions that had made her sick" (p. 63).

Betty expressed similar concerns when she described father's final public beating of her. She said she was "relieved to have adult witnesses so that someone finally would believe."

Erikson (1962) discusses the preoccupation with factual truth seen in late adolescence and young adulthood and states that this quest may be of "acute relevance to the ego's adaptive strength" (p. 458). Freud has been criticized by some (Erikson 1962; Jennings 1986; Krohn and Krohn 1982; Malcolm 1987; Marcus 1985) for minimizing the severity of Dora's abusive situation. However, others have pointed out that the only reason we know the horrible details of Dora's situation is because Freud carefully assembled them—the angry scenes between her parents about Frau K.; the awkward daily arrival of flowers from Herr K.; Dora's terror at age 13 (Dexter 1991) when she found herself struggling alone to escape Herr K.'s passionate embrace when she had believed that the purpose of the outing was to see a parade. Others have suggested, as with Anna O. (see Chapter 7) that actual father-daughter incest cannot be ruled out in this household, where Dora served as her father's nighttime nurse from age 8 (Bernstein 1989).

The literature in the field of child abuse and incest treatment (Goodwin 1985, 1988, 1990; Goodwin et al., in press; Steele 1986) emphasizes the importance of psychotherapy as an atmosphere of safety for the reconstruction of childhood trauma. Freud, too, emphasized the importance of restoring Dora's ability to form a connected, coherent intelligible narrative. One of us (Goodwin 1990) has recommended specific investigational interventions, including reviews of pediatric records; interviews by the patient of siblings and neighbors; and review of family photograph albums, diaries, and other materials. Confrontation and "apology" sessions with parent perpetrators are also recommended in selected situations.

Noncompliance

Freud struggled in his treatment of Dora, as we did in our eight cases, with perplexing issues of noncompliance. On one occasion, Dora obviously concealed a letter from her grandmother, as if to tease Freud. She was openly contemptuous of physicians. After Freud's interpretation of Dora's jewel case dream, he noted that Dora "would not follow this part of the interpretation" (1905/1971, p. 88). Indeed, it was at this point that Dora had made her silent decision to leave therapy. Dora was still angry about those dream interpretations when she met Felix Deutsch 24 years later (1957). In breaking off treatment abruptly 2 weeks later, she demonstrated her most defiant act of noncompliance. Freud took this behavior quite personally; " . . . this was an unmistakable act of vengeance on her part" (1905/1971, p. 131). Chart review indicated that some past treatments of our eight patients had failed when therapists viewed this noncompliance as a personal affront and insisted that it cease.

In Betty's case, we focused on helping her to deal with the pain of therapy without her having to stay away or fall asleep. In general, this was accomplished by our 5-minute review at the end of each session to look for where we may have "hit a nerve" and to anticipate difficulties in getting to the next session. On occasion a longer review was needed, such as after presentations of frightening dreams or discussions of her overwhelming rage. In these situations, she sometimes arranged a treat for herself after sessions; once she had a friend meet her to spirit her away from psychotherapy early. In addition, we anticipated for several weeks any disruptions in our scheduled appointments; holidays or visits to her mother were especially disruptive. Her need to control the psychotherapy became most clear when we could see it in parallel to her need to control her mother.

Reconstructing Parents

Betty's efforts to reconstruct her mother were quite self-conscious. She was less aware of how much she limited her feelings and statements in treatment because she experienced the therapist as someone just like her mother who had to be carefully handled and shielded from her emotions, especially her grief and anger. The imaginative reconstruction of the parents in reality and in therapy operates at many levels: first, to make it seem as if the child abuse never happened; then to make it seem as if there really are trustworthy parents and, by analogy, other trustworthy authority figures; and finally, to reduce the feelings of panic and rage that remain attached to memories of parental abuse. The problem, of course, is that this was not the reality; every effort to redesign the parent, no matter how ingenious, is doomed at one level to failure. Psychotherapy allows some learning from the failures.

Dora, too, was preoccupied with fixing or healing her father. She was also adept at constructing substitute mothers, such as her governess. For Dora, the K.'s had offered a substitute family with much of what was denied her at home—younger siblings, an intelligent and rational mother, and a healthy and attentive father. Given this view, it is easier to understand her disappointment and rage on realizing that her father's pathology and egoism (as well as her own pathology) reached even into this imaginary refuge.

Reconstructing and Completing Childhood

Betty actively kept herself in childhood. She watched children's programs, finger painted, took herself to see the *Nutcracker* every Christmas, and said "I'm not as old as other 28-year-olds." At age 28, still in college, she plans to work with children once she is finished. She became panicky when adult developmental issues surfaced—falling in love, marriage, having babies—and said "Once you're tied down with a husband and a kid, that's it, the fun is over."

Like Betty, Dora was trying to catch up on her childhood—attending lectures, trying to develop a courting relationship with a peer. Dora also seems to have tended to flee at those moments when Freud asked her to process adult material in an adult way. She said she made her decision to leave therapy at about the time when Freud so brilliantly analyzed her famous jewel case dream. Freud (1905/1971) interpreted the dream as expressing Dora's fears of yielding to her feelings of sexual love for Herr K. Marcus (1985) describes this line of Freud's interpretations as follows: "... he treats her throughout as if this fourteen-, sixteen-, and eighteen-year-old adolescent had the capacities for sexual response of a grown woman" (p. 78). By fleeing from therapy as she did, Dora may have been expressing to Freud what Betty has told me repeatedly: "I'm not ready for this."

Chronic Rage

Dora was brought into treatment because of "some really remarkable achievements in the direction of intolerable behavior" (Freud 1905/1971)—refusing to see the K.'s; leaving a suicide note for her father. When she finally did confront the K.'s, it was on the occasion of their child's death—another instance of "intolerable behavior."

When Felix Deutsch saw Dora in her middle age (1957), he described the "reproachful demands" she made of her husband and son, which "tortured" them. Freud and her brother were the only people in her life for whom she had a kind word. However, when the brother pled with Deutsch to take on Dora's case again, Deutsch declined—perhaps in part because he found her rageful behaviors "repulsive."

One of the problems with Freud's emphasis on Dora's sexuality was the relative slighting of her aggressive feelings. In the jewel case dream that she and Freud argued about so persistently, the house was on fire and Dora was wakened by her father. Her mother wanted to stop and save her jewel case. The father said "I refuse to let myself and my two children be burnt for the sake of your jewel case." Freud's interpretation emphasized Dora's fears of the internal sexual fires kindled in her by Herr K. Another way to see the dream would be as a statement of Dora's fear and frustration that her parents were so entangled in their individual and mutual pathologies that they literally would not be able to care well enough for her to save her from a fire, even an external fire. The futility of seeking parental guidance in coping with internal fires or moral dilemmas had already been amply demonstrated during the years when Dora's father had made her his willing but unwitting accomplice in his affair with Frau K. As Freud said (1905/1971), "Her father was himself partly responsible for her present danger for he had handed her over to this strange man in the interests of his own love affair" (p. 105). Dora's father was not a fireman so much as an arsonist.

Freud interpreted Dora's suicide note as an attempt to imitate her father's ploy of disguising his sexual liaisons with Frau K. as crisis intervention for his suicidality. However the suicidal thoughts together with Dora's multiple somatic symptoms, including shortness of breath, could also be understood as a communication that her very life was in danger. Her intermittent flooding with death fears may have conditioned her peremptory, demanding behaviors that might have seemed less obnoxious to Freud had he understood them as her desperate attempts to avoid threats that she perceived as potentially lethal, if not to her present survival, to her future happiness.

Betty found it even more difficult to talk about her rage than to describe her childhood abuse. It was 7 months before she confessed to violent acts in the past and then began to share her fantasies about getting revenge on her father and other people who had hurt her. The revenge fantasies conflicted so deeply with the dreams of reconstructing the parents that her aggression was sometimes completely split off and covered by amnesia.

What helped most in understanding Betty's rage was to connect its flare-ups with threats to her reconstructions of childhood and a better family. When her ballet class, her penny collection, her carefully choreographed visits to mother, or her reconstructed brother-boyfriends were threatened, Betty's rage became uncontrolled. As she recognized more and more how dangerous and miserable had been the real life that she was trying to improve through these imaginative reconstructions, she began to recognize the fear and sadness that lay beneath the anger.

Could Dora have been kept in treatment had Freud been able to make sense for Dora of what he termed her "malignant vindictiveness?" If Dora was like Betty, her carefully orchestrated manipulations of her surrogate family, the K.'s, and of her surrogate parent, Freud, were fueled by a desperate wish to avoid a repetition of the painful deception and abandonments she had experienced in childhood, and, beyond that, to make those old childhood wounds vanish entirely by creating the illusion that the hurts had never occurred.

Summary

Our reading of the rich material presented by Freud in the Dora case is only one of many possible. We focused on four major themes. First, Dora's vengeful noncompliance was such a problem that it led to Freud's first elaboration of the concept of transference. Second, Dora's main goal in treatment was to reform her parents and parent-figures—not (as Freud had hoped) to reform her own behavior. Third, Dora's interest in her own development was based on fears that she had been irreparably damaged by her parents and needs to redo childhood and adolescent tasks at a far earlier level than the sexual issues that Freud asked her to address. Fourth, Dora's somatic symptoms, suicidality, and "intolerable behavior" stemmed from her unresolved rage about her childhood neglect.

These same four themes were central in the psychotherapies of the eight young adult patients with child abuse histories who are described in this chapter. All presented compliance problems based on fear of repeated abuse in treatment. The only one not still heavily involved in reforming abusive parents had lost both parents to death. All were still working on adolescent and preadolescent developmental issues as reflected in their continuing identity as students and in the fact that only one had established an identity as head of household. Chronic rage was expressed directly in psychotherapy and indirectly through compliance problems. Six of the eight showed "intolerable behaviors" (i.e., some combination of violence to self or others, substance abuse, and eating disorders).

Psychotherapeutically, focusing on the child abuse seemed to provide a way out of the noncompliance problems; perhaps with longer term follow-up, this will prove helpful for the other elements of the syndrome. The patients' attempts to make the child abuse disappear by reconstructing parents, redoing childhood, and masking their rage as badness seem to continue endlessly and compulsively until the abuse can be remembered and grieved. At this point their development can be freed from the impossible task of exonerating or punishing their parents and can become the construction of their own lives rather than a never-satisfactory reconstruction of childhood.

References

Bernstein A: Analysis of two adult female patients who had been victims of incest in childhood. J Am Acad Psychoanal 17:207–221, 1989

Dexter H: Freud, Dora, and Vienna 1900. New York, Free Press, 1991

Deutsch F: A Footnote to Freud's "Fragment of an Analysis of a Case of Hysteria." Psychoanal Q 26:159–167, 1957

Erikson E: Reality and actuality: an address. J Am Psychoanal Assoc 10:451–474, 1962

Freud S: Dora: An Analysis of a Case of Hysteria (Fragment of an Analysis of a Case of Hysteria) (1905). Edited by Reiff P. New York, Collier Books, Macmillan, 1971

Goodwin J: Family violence: principles of intervention and prevention. Hosp Community Psychiatry 36:1074–1079, 1985

Goodwin J: Post-traumatic symptoms in abused children. Journal of Traumatic Stress 1:475–488, 1988

Goodwin J: Applying to adult incest victims what we have learned from victimized children, in The Adult Incest Victim. Edited by Kluft R. Washington, DC, American Psychiatric Press, 1990, pp 55–74

Goodwin J, Attias R, McCarty T, et al: Effects on psychiatric inpatients of routine questioning about childhood sexual abuse. Victimology (in press)

Jennings J: The revival of "Dora": advances in psychoanalytic theory and technique. J Am Psychoanal Assoc 34:607–635, 1986

Krohn A, Krohn J: The nature of the Oedipus complex in the Dora case. J Am Psychoanal Assoc 30:555–578, 1982

Mai T: Representation of patriarchy: sexuality and epistemology in Freud's Dora, in In Dora's Case: Freud-Hysteria-Feminism. Edited by Bernheimer C, Kahane C. New York, Columbia University Press, 1985, pp 181–199

Malcolm J: Reflections: J'appelle un chat un chat. The New Yorker, April 20, 1987, pp 84–102

Marcus S: Freud and Dora: story, history, case history, in In Dora's Case: Freud-Hysteria-Feminism. Edited by Bernheimer C, Kahane C. New York, Columbia University Press, 1985, pp 56–91

Sprengnether M: Enforcing Oedipus: Freud and Dora, in In Dora's Case: Freud-Hysteria-Feminism. Edited by Bernheimer C, Kahan C. New York, Columbia University Press, 1985, pp 254–275

Steele F: Child abuse, in The Reconstruction of Trauma: Its Significance in Clinical Work (Workshop Series). Edited by Rothstein A. Madison, CT, International Universities Press, 1986, pp 59–72

Section VI

A Modern Psychoanalytic Case

> We are healed of a suffering only by experiencing it to the full.
>
> Marcel Proust, *Remembrance of Things Past*

> I want to talk about my tragic story because if I don't, it will get into my mind and into my dream and make me crazy. I know some people died of their tragic story.
>
> Gus Bighorse, Navajo elder
> *Bighorse the Warrior*

> It is my impression that the most productive and creative lives are lived by those who, despite high degrees of traumatization in childhood, are able to . . . find new routes toward inner completeness.
>
> Heinz Kohut
> *The Restoration of the Self*

Editor's Introduction

Ever since the Greeks gave us Orestes pursued by the tormenting Furies, we have known that traumatic experience can lead at times to madness. The folklore of possession and exorcism describes people speaking in many different voices, sometimes attacking their caretakers, violently resisting restraint, and experiencing a variety of physical symptoms, including bizarre eating disorders (see Chapter 4).

Freud described the case of Daniel Paul Schreber, a middle-aged judge who became depressed and suicidal and was committed to a psychiatric hospital where his behavior became frankly psychotic. Schreber believed he was being tied down by rays from God and that his body was being touched in sexually tormenting ways. Later research by Niederland (1959) revealed that Schreber's father, a prominent pediatrician, had invented devices to control children's posture and had used these to break the child's spirit. He had also employed pedagogic techniques, such as having young Daniel write down his infractions and then request punishment (his son in his psychosis was to depict this last as the "writing down miracle"). Schreber's only brother died by suicide. Schreber's symptoms are precisely those we would expect in a victim of extreme childhood abuse: self-mutilation and suicidality, depression, dissociative episodes to the point of catatonia, immersion in fantasy and the past, eating disorder, angry outbursts, provocations of reabuse, and a litany of perplexing somatic symptoms (Goodwin et al. 1990). More recent reviewers (de Mause 1987) have speculated that forced sodomy and fellatio in addition to physical abuse could have been elements of the traumatic childhood situation that were translated into those of Schreber's delusions, which concerned being seduced and turned into a woman by God.

Wolf Man, the other of Freud's cases who sustained multiple hospitalizations and recurrent suicidality, came from a family like Schreber's, where there was a troubled and at times psychotic parent and where one sibling (the patient's incestuous partner) had already committed suicide. As in present-day cases, the clustering suggests that it is the raw extremity of the abuse situation, more than some inherent weakness in the victim, that leads to psychotic levels of symptoms.

This link between trauma and madness was rediscovered in an elegant paper by van der Kolk (1987). A middle-aged woman became psychotic while nursing her dying father. She felt that gases and electricity were invading her body, and she had become preoccupied with Nazis. She approached strangers asking "How many did you save?" Her most disruptive symptoms involved setting off fire alarms and marching her fellow patients out of the hospital. What underlay all this was her experience, more than 30 years previously, of the Coconut Grove nightclub fire, a disastrous fire in 1942 that killed almost 500 people. The fire was a landmark for psychiatry, because it led to Lindemann's (1944) classic studies on grief and to his interpersonal definition of trauma as the sudden cessation of social interaction. Each one of this woman's symptoms could be linked to some aspect of this fire, which began in electrical wiring, poisoned the air in the nightclub, and led to the blocking of the main exit door by bodies. In addition, this woman's experience of polio in early childhood had provided the dissociative structures that determined the course of her later traumatic responses in late adolescence and mid-adulthood.

The case described in the next chapter also involves severe symptoms: self-mutilation with anesthesia, conversion pain, conversion blindness, a complex delusional world, voices giving commands to self-harm, and delusional guilt. *I Never Promised You A Rose Garden,* published in 1964 under the pseudonym of Hannah Green, is one of a growing library of memoirs of illness written by former patients (Sommer and Osmond 1983). Joanne Greenberg (1964/1981), who has now claimed the classic as her own work (Rubin 1972), was treated by Frieda Fromm-Reichmann at Chestnut Lodge from 1948 to 1952. In those 4 years of analytic treatment, Fromm-Reichmann and the patient unraveled the connections between these florid symptoms and the extensive medical trauma in early childhood that had schooled Joanne in escapes into fantasy.

In retrospect, Fromm-Reichmann was deploying many techniques described previously in this book. Her instinct for good psychotherapeutic technique encompassed trauma as it did so many other areas of treatment. Having worked for the Prussian Army in her youth (caring for soldiers brain-damaged in World War I), Fromm-Reichmann was not afraid of confrontation. She told her patient to tell her gods:

> I don't like them, tell them I don't believe in them, tell them I think they're keeping you from everything that's good and valuable, tell them we're at war. Make no apology for that. I'm not on their side. I'm on your side. (Silver 1989, p. 518)

No folk exorcist could have framed more clearly the battle lines being drawn around the introjected abusers. Fromm-Reichmann also understood that the patient had to become a chief architect of the therapeutic bridge he or she was building toward health. Like Despine, she took the patient's advice seriously. She respected the patient's need for symptoms and promised not to take away Deborah's "darling" self-mutilations until the patient was ready. Like Freud with Dora, Fromm-Reichmann insisted on a full narrative of each aspect of the situation and used collateral data to resolve discrepancies. She fought dissociative amnesia for the treatment sessions by introducing end-of-session summaries (see Chapter 8).

In these patients with histories of massive medical trauma in early childhood, a clinician faces many dilemmas when psychotic-level posttraumatic symptoms call for hospitalization. For patients like Estelle, Deborah Blau, and van der Kolk's childhood polio victim, the hospital is critical for protection and for maintaining basic bodily functions but is at the same time a minefield of triggers for retraumatization. Separation from home, enforced incarceration, use of isolation and restraint, intrusive medical procedures, rigid schedules, symptoms of illness in peers—all are experienced as overwhelming repetitions in a self-system regressed to preoperational developmental levels. For some of these patients, the emotional costs of hospitalization may outweigh the benefits of increased safety and intensity of treatment. Many of Deborah Blau's episodes of self-harm seemed to occur when intrusive aspects of hospital routine stirred up powerful feelings and impulses too intense to be understood and neutralized by psychotherapy in time to prevent enactment (Favazza and Favazza 1987). For the future, if we are to treat such individuals without creating iatrogenic crises, we need to design intensive day programs and inpatient facilities stripped as much as possible of the pseudomilitary trappings of medicine and reformed as true refuges and asylums.

I still recall my first encounter with *Rose Garden.* In the 1960s, as today, one came to the book on the basis of word-of-mouth recommendation. It was an all night, can't-put-it-down read back then; and even now that I know this terrain so well, it remains an absolutely gripping account of the painful work that waits to be done in these cases where trauma has been so profoundly shattering to the self.

References

deMause L: Schreber and the history of childhood. Journal of Psychohistory 15:424–430, 1987

Favazza AR, Favazza B: Bodies Under Siege: Self-Mutilation in Culture and Psychiatry. Baltimore, MD, Johns Hopkins University Press, 1987

Goodwin J, Cheeves K, Connell V: Borderline and other severe symptoms in adult survivors of incestuous abuse. Psychiatric Annals 20:22–32, 1990

Greenberg J (Green H): I Never Promised You a Rose Garden (1964). New York, Holt Rinehart & Winston, 1981

Lindemann E: Symptomatology and management of acute grief. Am J Psychiatry 101:141–148, 1944

Niederland WG: Schreber, father and son. Psychoanal Q 28:151–169, 1959

Rubin SE: Conversations with the author of "I Never Promised You a Rose Garden." Psychoanal Rev 59:201–215, 1972

Silver AL: Psychoanalysis and Psychosis. Madison, CT, International Universities Press, 1989

Sommer R, Osmond H: A bibliography of mental patients' autobiographies. Am J Psychiatry 140:1051–1054, 1983 van der Kolk B: Amnesia, dissociation, and the return of the repressed, in Psychological Trauma. Edited by van der Kolk B. Washington, DC, American Psychiatric Press, 1987, pp 173–190

Chapter 9

I Never Promised You a Rose Garden: Compulsive Self-Mutilation

Barbara J. Murray, M.D.

Self-mutilating behaviors are noted in DSM-III-R (American Psychiatric Association 1987) in only five diagnostic categories—borderline personality disorder, multiple personality disorder, sexual masochism, factitious disorder, and trichotillomania (American Psychiatric Association 1987). Such behaviors are present in most patients diagnosed as having a major dissociative disorder. Ross (1989) studied 236 cases of multiple personality disorder and found self-inflicted injuries present in 56.6% of the subjects and wrist-slashing in 49.3%. Within this diagnostic group, parasuicidal behaviors were associated with higher levels of prior physical and sexual abuse. Self-mutilating behavior is reported more commonly in women, usually starting in adolescence, with peak incidence occurring between the ages of 15 to 35. Often, a history of sexual and/or physical abuse is found. Favazza (1989) found 62% of females who were self-mutilators gave a history of childhood physical and/or sexual abuse. Typical self-mutilating behaviors include cutting the body, burning with cigarettes or caustic substances, banging heads and arms against walls, swallowing poisons or overdoses of medication, and mutilating genitalia.

Numerous theories have been suggested to explain the compulsion to self-mutilate:

1. Physical pain as a way of distracting oneself from or releasing severe emotional pain, depression, anxiety, or anger;
2. A release from guilt or a need for self-punishment;
3. Attention-seeking behavior to relieve loneliness;

4. An action over which one has complete control, unlike other areas in one's life;
5. For those experiencing physical or emotional numbness, a stimulation to the body that makes one feel alive;
6. An unconscious urge to disfigure oneself and make oneself less likely to be viewed as a sexual being, and therefore less likely to be sexually assaulted;
7. To enhance or dampen sexual feelings; and
8. A response to command hallucinations (Favazza 1989; Favazza and Conterio 1989).

Dissociative experiences often accompany self-mutilating behavior. The trancelike states of depersonalization and derealization, frequently with a lack of feeling of pain and partial amnesia, are often interrupted by the self-destructive act, with subsequent return to awareness. The sense of lack of control of behavior in dissociation and confusion caused by different ego states can lead to self-mutilating behaviors.

The following cases illustrate the diagnostic problems in two cases of self-mutilating behaviors accompanied by dissociation. The first case "Deborah," is drawn from the 1964 autobiographical novel *I Never Promised You a Rose Garden,* which describes a girl diagnosed as "schizophrenic" and treated by Frieda Fromm-Reichmann in the late 1940s and early 1950s (Greenberg 1964/1981). The person in the second case, "Ann," whose case is presented here because of its remarkable similarities to the first, was treated in a rural community mental health center in the 1980s.

Case Study 1—Deborah

Deborah Blau of *I Never Promised You a Rose Garden* was hospitalized at the age of 16 with a diagnosis of schizophrenia, after she made a suicide attempt by cutting her wrist.

Deborah was the oldest of two children born to a first-generation American family. Her maternal grandfather, who was Latvian and Jewish, played a key role in her early years and was the primary provider for the family. Deborah's mother grew up realizing that all of the financial success and culture that her father tried to bring to them were futile because a prejudiced world viewed their family with contempt. When blonde Deborah was born, she was viewed as a golden child in her grandfather's eyes. Deborah had various nurses and governesses caring for her. When she was quite young, her mother had a miscarriage and "went away to rest" for a while. As Deborah recalled it, "everything warm had left," (p. 98) and she was left with a cold and distant nurse.

Around age 5, Deborah began to have problems with urinary incontinence. Her rigid governesses became "righteously wrathful" because her incontinence could not be cured by shaming "or whipping or threats" (p. 36). It was only after numerous medical evaluations that a urethral tumor was diagnosed. Deborah described a sense of "wrongness inside her in the feminine part" (p. 44). She recalled that probes and needles were used "as if the entire reality of her body were concentrated in the secret evil inside that forbidden place" (p. 44). She felt the doctors lied to her, promising her nothing would hurt. She had vivid memories of the "searing stroke of the instrument" and remembered a doctor saying that he was going to put her doll to sleep as they lowered the ether mask over her. Then followed "the hardest, longest, burning of that secret place" that she could imagine. She had memories of being tied to a table with doctors saying things such as "we are going to fix you fine now" (p. 45). She was sure that they were going to murder her. They never said they were sorry or apologized to her for the trauma.

Deborah believed that she never quite lost the tumor; this became the seed of her sense of being poisonous to those in her life, describing herself as having "Deborah rot." She had two surgical procedures in a short time. During this time, her mother was also pregnant with her sister, who was born shortly after Deborah's surgery. Because of health problems, Deborah started school late and did not feel accepted by her peer group and was often the target of anti-Semitic remarks. She was sent to summer camp from the ages of 6 through 9, a camp that unbeknownst to her parents was strongly anti-Semitic. She never told her parents the cruelty she experienced there, but her mother noted when Deborah was about 9 that "something went out of her. It was as if she had her head down from then on awaiting for the blows" (p. 42). She appeared to be an unhappy, clumsy, and extremely intense young girl. She turned to compulsive overeating for comfort. Insomnia became a constant problem. Several moves occurred in the next few years because of financial instability in the family, making it very difficult for Deborah to develop any stable peer relationships. She was viewed by her family as the special golden child, but in her peer world, she was ignored and abused.

Deborah became aware of some of her father's unconscious incestuous feelings and fantasies. She saw him as always trying to make her frightened of men, describing scenes of men lurking behind trees and bushes, intending to grab her from dark streets. He talked to her of sex maniacs and thieves. He let her know that he believed men were brutes and animals, lusting without limits. On one occasion, she saw an exhibitionist on the street, and her father believed that she must have done something to encourage him and scolded her severely for this.

Deborah noted that often she was rebuffed or yelled at for things she had no memories of doing. Maids left their home because she would not apologize, but she never knew for what or why. Friends would turn a cold shoulder to her and she never knew why, but they clearly implied she had done or said something offensive to them, suggesting that she was losing time.

It was during the years at the anti-Semitic camp that Deborah developed the kingdom of Yr. Yr contained several "gods" who spoke a special language—Anterrabae, Lactamaeon, and Idat—a "Collect" of derisive, critical voices, a "Censor," and a Japanese soldier. In between the world and Yr was a transition zone called the mid world. Yr had a neutral place called the fourth level where "there was no emotion to endure, no past or future to grind against, no memory or possession of self, nothing except dead facts which came unbidden when she needed them and which had no feeling attached to them" (p. 11). Her entry into Yr was often heralded by loss of vision, loss of hearing, anesthesia, and shivering. Initially, the gods were comforting but became more demanding as the years went on. She often was caught in between the collision of the world of Yr and the world of reality. Yr was described as having "golden meadows and Gods" and also "regions of horror and lostness" (p. 16). The gods often sent her signs or omens.

Shortly before her 16th birthday, Deborah went to her doctor for recurrent abdominal pain. Recalling that day, she "realized she had lost another day" (p. 63). She was found by her mother, sitting on the bathroom floor quietly watching her blood from her cut wrist flow into a basin. She stated she had not wanted the blood to get too far away from her and realized that she was not attempting to commit suicide but making a call for help. It was at this point that she was hospitalized.

(The author's hospitalization was at Chestnut Lodge and her treating psychiatrist was Frieda Fromm-Reichmann.)

Evaluation at the hospital revealed Deborah to be a bright woman with an IQ of 140 to 150 who was diagnosed as having schizophrenia with strong compulsive and masochistic components. She was treated in intensive psychotherapy and confined to the hospital for several years. Her treatment was punctuated with marked conflict between the world of the gods and the world of reality. The world of the gods described a dissociated state in which she would lose large amounts of time. She carried out frequent self-mutilating behaviors. On one occasion, she took the top of a tin can and made several deep cuts in her arm, feeling no pain. There were also cigarette burns to her arms. At times she would be found beating her head against tiled floors. In seclusion rooms, Deborah was seen hurling herself across the room, hitting her head and body on the walls. In addition to psychotherapy because of her major behavioral problems, Deborah was given psychotropic medications as well as icy cold wet packs to subdue her. Slowly, she built a trusting relationship with her therapist; she was able to assume more control of her life with eventual but slow recovery through intensive insight-oriented psychotherapy. In therapy, the gods of Yr were traced to illustrations of falling angels from *Paradise Lost,* a book strongly associated with her grandfather and her childhood perceptions of his myths about himself and Deborah. The Japanese soldier, too, was connected to her grandfather's stubborn pride, stoicism, and foreignness and to her childhood fantasies about World War II as a macrocosmic mirror of her personal conflicts. The Collect and Censor had arisen to insulate these problematic identifications from each other and from her everyday life.

Case Study 2—Ann

Ann, a 22-year-old college student, was referred by her outpatient therapist for psychiatric evaluation of thought disturbances and possible hallucinations. She had a history of two previous hospitalizations for anorexia, explaining that her parents were not involved in her treatment because "they felt it was my problem, not theirs and they felt they would be blamed for my problems if they came." She felt her family was "sick of me and they don't understand my problem." She admitted to feeling confused most of the time. She denied feeling depressed; however, clinically she presented a picture of chronic depression. She had intermittent thoughts of suicide and a history of suicidal gestures. She complained of feeling like "my brain shuts down." She felt time seemed to speed up or slow down for her, and she lost track of where she was with some of her school projects. It was hard for her to focus on people's conversations; roommates avoided her, because they found her odd. She often heard her name being called but also on occasion heard "rapid conversations I could not understand." She believed her grandfather was able to control her thoughts and put thoughts into her mind and that she could read others' minds.

Ann was the second of six children and had three sisters and two brothers. She had few memories of her early years. School records noted she was shy and quiet, that it took her several months to develop confidence each school year, and that she often appeared confused. An eighth-grade teacher noted she always looked like she wanted to cry and was under a lot of tension. Her father was a social worker who was described as a constricted man, unable to express much emotion. Her mother worked as a teacher and was seen by Ann as perfectionistic and highly critical.

Ann's overt psychiatric problems began in the ninth grade. She fractured her arm in an accident, missed some school, fell behind in her schoolwork, and felt overwhelmed. She began some wrist scratching and cutting at this time. The school became increasingly concerned about suicidal thoughts that she confided to school friends and notified the family. Ann was hospitalized for the first time at age 14. Testing revealed a major learning disability and average IQ; in a family of high achievers, this was considered a major failing for Ann. Projective testing revealed that Ann was sad and lonely, making frequent use of a fantasy world. She viewed her parents as vigilant, demanding, and patronizing. She perceived herself as being odd and different from others.

Her depression was severe and pervasive. Ann showed morbid preoccupation with death and dying, working very hard to appear controlled on the surface while underneath there was chaos and helplessness. Her diagnosis was major affective disorder, depressed with psychotic features. She was hospitalized for 3 months and made frequent attempts at suicide, requiring physical restraint and neuroleptic medication. Ann's eating disorder behaviors began at age 15, with more extreme caloric restriction emerging in college, together with excessive exercise, laxative abuse, and self-induced vomiting, which led to hospitalization. Her diagnoses at discharge were atypical eating disorder with dysthymia and anxiety disorder. During one of the hospitalizations for the eating disorder, Ann complained of "occasional mental lapses." Neurological evaluation demonstrated no organic pathology.

In therapy in college, Ann admitted that she had been physically and verbally abused by a sister who she believed was being sexually abused by their grandfather. She stated that this sister often would be laughing at and mocking her as she hit. Ann also believed that her mother was verbally cruel and abusive toward her. Ann initially denied that she had been sexually abused. Only much later during a lengthy hospitalization did she recall and reveal that an uncle, a Protestant minister, sexually abused her over several years.

Attempts were made to treat Ann on an outpatient basis while she was in college. She began to confide to her therapists about her world of the gods. Initially, the gods had been soothing and helpful; but as the years went by, they became more punitive. At times she felt safer in the world of the gods. She noted that the gods were giving her frequent messages. They would give her "landmarks" to tell her if her day was going to be good and these "landmarks" were often common things she would see in her environment, such as a license plate or a particular color car, giving her special indications about how the gods were feeling about her. In the course of therapy, Ann identified one of the voices of the gods as her father's; another god, described as the "laughing god," had her sister's voice.

The gods were extremely powerful; Ann would say "[they] force me to do things against my will" such as failing exams, losing a job, and getting involved in eating disorder behaviors. In therapy, she began to connect these gods with her uncle's threats of divine punishment if she did not obey him. A diagnosis of dissociative disorder versus posttraumatic stress disorder with dissociative symptoms was made. Frequent major crises, including abuse of a babysitting charge, increasing suicide potential, a near-lethal overdose, and malnutrition from the eating disorder finally necessitated Ann's hospitalization.

Ann's admitting diagnoses to a long-term institution were atypical psychosis and atypical eating disorder. Neuroleptic, antidepressant, and antianxiety medications as well as ECT were used unsuccessfully in her treatment. Intensive psychotherapy was the primary mode of treatment. However, as the memories of more extensive and brutal abuse surfaced, behavioral management became a prime concern. Ann made almost daily suicide attempts and attempted self-abusive and assaultive behaviors. She made frequent attempts to mutilate her face, gouge her eyes out, and bang her head, as well as attempts at strangling herself with shoelaces or telephone or television wires, cutting, self-electrocution, suffocation, and inhalation of various substances.

Ultimately, Ann required round-the-clock restraints with two or three staff members by her side constantly. Despite this, she succeeded in completing suicide. Ann's final diagnoses included posttraumatic stress disorder, dissociative disorder not otherwise specified, mixed personality disorder, and anorexia nervosa.

Conclusion

Both cases discussed in this chapter involve self-mutilation, fantasy worlds, auditory hallucinations, eating disorders, sensory losses, and lost time with amnesia. Deborah Blau clearly gave a history of physical trauma associated with medical care and emotional and probably physical abuse by nurses and governesses, rejection and probable abuse by peers because of her Jewish background, and possible covert incestuous themes in her relationship with her father. Her slow but clear response to intensive psychotherapy is not supportive of a diagnosis of schizophrenia but perhaps of posttraumatic stress disorder and dissociative disorder, similar to the picture of Ann in the second case study. Ann was also diagnosed at various times with primary psychotic disorders such as schizoaffective disorder and schizophrenia. Uncovering this contemporary patient's physical and sexual abuse in childhood clarified the posttraumatic origins of her florid symptoms.

Schneiderian symptoms, or delusions of control, which were present in both these cases, have been recognized recently as more characteristic of multiple personality disorder than of schizophrenia (Kluft 1987).

Although dissociative episodes were disabling in both cases, multiple personality disorder could not be documented. As in cases of "possession" (see Chapters 3 and 4), in these two cases, the imagined protective identities remained at the level of imaginary companions rather than becoming enacted as self-fragments. Deborah and Ann both found their world of gods comforting at first but then increasingly frightening and controlling. "Laughing gods" embodied aspects of the malevolent childhood contexts (Gelinas 1991) that involved being ridiculed. Having fled the real world as too painful, they found their new imaginary worlds increasingly peopled by introjects of the various abusers they had striven to escape.

In summary, a historical case commonly thought to illustrate schizophrenia has been reviewed and rediagnosed in light of increasing awareness of the sequelae of childhood trauma and the growing knowledge of the role of dissociation in abuse victims. Self-mutilating behaviors are often a sequelae of child abuse histories and, when present, should lead to screening for posttraumatic or dissociative diagnoses. The long process described in *Rose Garden* of protective care and intensive interpretation seems still to map the treatment of choice in such cases.

References

American Psychiatric Association: Diagnostic and Statistical Manual of Mental Disorders, 3rd Edition, Revised. Washington, DC, American Psychiatric Association, 1987

Favazza AR: Why patients mutilate themselves. Hosp Community Psychiatry 40:137–145, 1989

Favazza AR, Conterio K: Female habitual self-mutilators. Acta Psychiatr Scand 79:283–289, 1989

Gelinas D: Traumas of malevolent intent: recognition, effects and intervention. Paper presented at the 7th annual convention of the International Society for Traumatic Stress Studies, Washington, DC, October 24–27, 1991

Greenberg J (Green H): I Never Promised You a Rose Garden (1964). New York, Holt Rinehart & Winston, 1981

Kluft RP: First-rank symptoms as a diagnostic clue to Multiple Personality Disorder. Am J Psychiatry 144:293–298, 1987

Ross C: Multiple Personality Disorder: Diagnosis, Clinical Features, and Treatment. New York, Wiley, 1989

Index

Page numbers in **boldface** *type refer to tables or figures.*